WALL PILATES

FOR SENIORS

Fully **Illustrated Workout Plan** for Reclaiming **Strength**,
Restoring **Balance**,
and Achieving **Weight Loss** in Just
28 Days

FitLife Solutions – Grow Your Health

PAGE 2

Table of Contents

About the Author

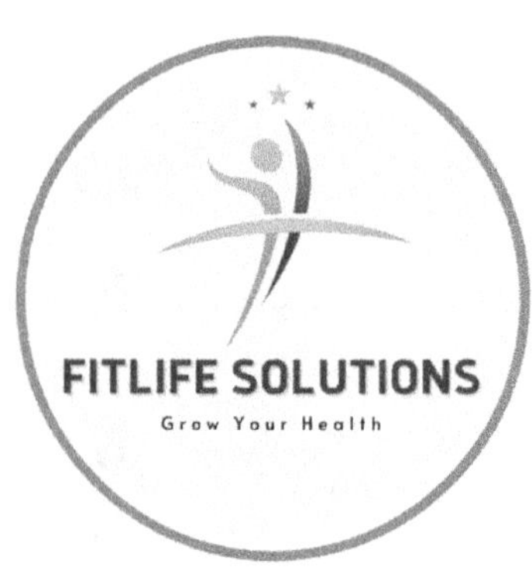

FitLife Solutions is a leading provider of fitness programs tailored to individuals of all ages and diverse needs. Our mission is to empower people to live healthier, happier lives through personalized fitness solutions.

At FitLife Solutions, we understand unique fitness goals and requirements and, therefore, offer a wide range of programs designed to cater to the specific needs of each individual. Whether you're a busy professional looking for more efficient workouts, an individual who has specialized fitness needs, or a senior wanting to improve flexibility and mobility, there's a program just for you.

Our team of certified trainers and experienced fitness experts work effortlessly to develop innovative, effective workout plans for the highest level of effectiveness, safety, and enjoyment. The latest research in exercise science is combined with practical, real-world applications when we create programs that deliver tangible results.

At FitLife Solutions, we strongly believe fitness is for everyone, regardless of ability, age, or background. We make fitness accessible, enjoyable, and rewarding for everyone, and we support you along your journey to better health and wellness.

Introduction

Welcome to Wall Pilates for Seniors. This book offers a complete guide to the powerful, yet gentle practice of Wall Pilates specifically targeting senior readers.

When we get older, keeping a level of balance, strength, and flexibility is important for our overall health. With Wall Pilates, we have crafted a safe and effective approach to exercise that addresses the unique needs and concerns of seniors.

Throughout these pages, you will discover a transformative 28-day workout plan. With just 15 minutes a day, this plan is created to change your life, providing a way to improve balance, strength, and vitality.

No matter if you are new to Pilates or an experienced pro, Wall Pilates for Seniors has something for you. What are you waiting for? Get your mat, and let's start on the path toward balance, strength, and vitality for the best years of your life.

Here's to a healthier, happier you!
FitLife Solutions Team

Special Bonus Offer!

Hello Readers,

You are a valued member of our fitness community, so we're excited to offer a wonderful bonus to help you on your path to fitness! Simply scan the **QR code** or **click on the link below**, and you'll be directed to our supplementary **Workout Progress Journal.**

QR code:

or **link:** <u>Workout Progress Journal</u>

The journal will assist you along your way toward fitness by providing a means to track your workouts, set individual goals, and monitor the progress you are making. The easy-to-use format and comprehensively-designed journal is a great tool to keep you on track, motivated, and accountable as you reach your fitness goals.

Don't miss out on this incredible opportunity to take your fitness journey to the next level.

Happy training,
FitLife Solutions Team

What is Wall Pilates?

Wall Pilates is a great way to get moving by using only a Mat and a wall nearby. It's different from Traditional Pilates which requires other props and equipment and is mostly performed in a class format. Wall Pilates only uses the wall's resistance and your body weight.

Specifically, in Wall Pilates, you use your feet, arms, sides, and back to press up against a wall while practicing many types of exercises including planks and squats. Your body weight and the wall add resistance against gravity.

It is perfect for those beginning to exercise or others who need more stability (while exercising). That's one reason it's so popular in senior living communities. Wall Pilates for Seniors targets older adults, combining traditional Pilates movements that yield so many benefits with added wall support.

Wall Pilates exercises focus on several key areas: strengthening core muscles, improving balance and posture, and boosting overall health and wellness.

First developed by Joseph Pilates in 1926 as a way to rehabilitate wounded soldiers, Pilates changed into a popular way of exercising for those wanting to improve overall health/fitness.

In summary, Wall Pilates is an effective and safe way to exercise for the senior population. With a focus on strengthening core muscles, improving balance and posture, and boosting overall health/wellness, it's a wonderful choice for those looking to improve their fitness and remain independent as they age. Wall Pilates, with its many benefits, is an exercise worth learning more about for anyone, especially seniors, who want to be active and stay healthy for the years to come.

Benefits of Wall Pilates Exercises for Seniors

Wall Pilates is an effective way to exercise for the senior population because it integrates slow, controlled movements, rather than high-intensity activities. This makes it much easier to understand and perform than many other forms of exercise.

The slow, controlled movements are an easy way for older individuals to benefit from physical activity, without putting undue strain on their bodies.

So if you're 60 years old or older and you want a way to remain active without overextending yourself, then give senior Wall Pilates a chance! It just might be what you are looking for.

There are many benefits of Wall Pilates for Seniors:

 **Enhanced Stability and Balance:** Throughout the aging process, maintaining balance is even more important in helping prevent injuries and falls. Wall Pilates increases the body's balance and proprioception while enhancing stability and coordination. Seniors can reduce the risk of falls and improve their balance by practicing these exercises.

 **Improved Strength and Flexibility:** The core muscles critical for stability and balance, including the back, abdominals, and pelvic floor are the focus of the exercises. Routine practice can help increase muscle strength and flexibility, impacting better posture and overall body control.

Benefits of Wall Pilates Exercises for Seniors

 **Enhanced Joint Health:** The low-impact and controlled aspect of Wall Pilates exercises is easy on the joints and appropriate for those with joint pain or arthritis. Routine practice can help with circulation, stiffness, and joint movement.

 **Improved Posture:** The exercises promote spinal support and proper alignment, helping develop better posture in time. Wall Pilates can help with the discomfort of poor posture and as the risk of spinal issues diminishes.

 **Contributes to Overall Well-being:** Routine practices can add to overall emotional resilience, mental clarity, and physical health. It inspires the senior population to be more active in their overall health and the aging process. This, in turn, greatly enhances the quality of life.

 **Adaptability and Customization:** The exercises can be modified quite easily for those who have various abilities, limitations with mobility, and chronic conditions. Participants can tailor their practice to any of their needs and move forward at their own pace.

 **Connects the Mind and Body:** Wall Pilates allows seniors to focus on their mindful movement, body awareness, and breath. This promotes a powerful mind-body connection, increasing stress reduction, relaxation, and overall mental well-being.

Wall Pilates and Its Principles

Wall Pilates uses the same six key principles as Pilates which are as follows:

1 ▶ Breathing

Throughout every Pilates exercise, your breath is coordinated with movement to maximize the workouts. Breathing is extremely important to most of the exercises.

2 ▶ Center

In Pilates, a lot of attention and focus are placed on the center of the body. The center of the body is the area between your public bone and lower ribs. The pelvic floor muscles and core are instrumental to the Pilates' movements. With a focus on the body center, you will be more able to engage, activate, and relax your pelvic floor muscles and core.

3 ▶ Concentration

Pilates exercises are about concentrating on every exercise to perform it in the best way and gain the most from it. Through concentration, you focus on the specific exercise and increase more acute body awareness.

4 ▶ Control

All of the exercises are performed in a conscious, deliberate, and controlled manner. In other words, no body part is left to its own devices! It is thought when you move with intention, you get greater value from the exercise.

5 **Flow**

When observing any Pilates workout session, you'll be certain to see the movements executed in a flow-like way. The idea behind this is that the exercise connects all body parts, beginning with the core, and then flowing throughout the body.

6 **Precision**

Increased body awareness is promoted in every movement. The exercises executed in a precise way ensure the appropriate alignment and placement with other body parts. Therefore, it's crucial to focus on making your form and technique perfect to reduce poor habits and patterns from any previous exercise.

Wall Pilates' Safety Tips and Precautions

- Before beginning an exercise program, **consulting with a healthcare professional** is recommended, especially when there are preexisting physical limitations and medical conditions.

- **Regularly warm up** your body prior to engaging in Pilates to prepare your musculature and reduce the risk of injury. Then make sure to **cool down** after the workout. Every workout following the plan starts with a warm-up and concludes with stretching. Make sure you follow this advice.

- **Avoid pain-causing exercises:** If there is any pain or discomfort from the specific exercise, stop exercising right away, adapt the exercise, or select a different movement that is more fitting for you.

- **Take breaks and stay hydrated:** Make sure to take breaks on a regular basis to rest and have time to recover, specifically if you are winded. Remember to drink enough water prior to, during, and after the exercise session so you are well-hydrated.

- **Listen to what your body says:** How does your body feel while exercising? How does it feel after exercising? If there is any discomfort or you are feeling any unusual symptoms, stop the Pilates exercises and, if necessary, seek medical advice.

By following these precautions and safety tips, seniors can reap the benefits of Wall Pilates and minimize the risk of injury. Safety is a priority; listen to what your body tells you throughout the entire workout session.

Breathing

Breathing plays a critical role in Wall Pilates. It increases the impact of the exercises and promotes relaxation.

Here's how breathing is typically incorporated into Wall Pilates:

Diaphragmatic breathing: Deep diaphragmatic breathing is known as belly breathing. This type of breathing is characterized by inhaling deeply through the nose, letting the belly expand, and exhaling completely through the mouth, pulling the belly button toward the spine. Diaphragmatic breathing involves the diaphragm, increases relaxation, and provides stability throughout the exercises.

Breath coordination: In Wall Pilates, breathing is coordinated with movement. It enhances control and flow. Usually, you inhale at the beginning of an exercise and exhale when performing the exertion or movement. This helps effectively engage the core muscles and maintain stability all through the movement.

Mindful breathing: With every Wall Pilates practice, the emphasis is on mindful breathing. Individuals focus their attention on the breathing sensations flowing in and out of the body. This technique of being mindful during exercises helps to sharpen awareness, diminish stress, and increase the mind-body connection.

Breathing

Rhythmic breathing: When conducting the exercises, there is often a rhythmic pattern of equal time for inhaling and exhaling. This pattern helps regulate the movement of the exercises, synchronize the movement with breath, and promote mindfulness.

Breathing in Wall Pilates is a central aspect of facilitating mindfulness, relaxation, proper alignment, and core engagement. Individuals should strive to maintain breath awareness while exercising to maximize their benefits.

These items are typically needed:

☑ **A wall:** Any wall space that offers sufficient room for movement and stretching comfortably will work.

☑ **An exercise/yoga mat:** Use a mat to support and cushion your body when doing stretches and floor exercises.

☑ **Comfortable clothing:** Wear stretchy, breathable clothing to allow freedom of movement. Stay away from clothing that's too loose or tight.

☑ **A water bottle:** Keeping a water bottle full and nearby helps you stay hydrated every step of the workout.

☑ **A towel:** To wipe away any sweat and keep more comfortable throughout the workout, a towel is suggested.

☑ **Positive mindset:** Like most things, a positive attitude along with the willingness to challenge yourself will add more benefits to your exercise sessions. Listen to what your body is saying and adapt the exercises to best meet your abilities and fitness levels.

Types of Exercises: Warm-Ups

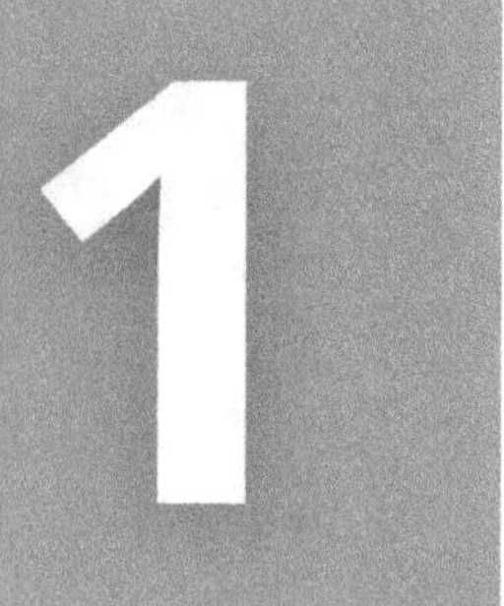

Wall Side Bends (Right, Left)

Wall Side Bends are ideal for warming up and stretching your external oblique abdominal muscles and the latissimus dorsi muscle (the large flat muscle in the lower thorax).

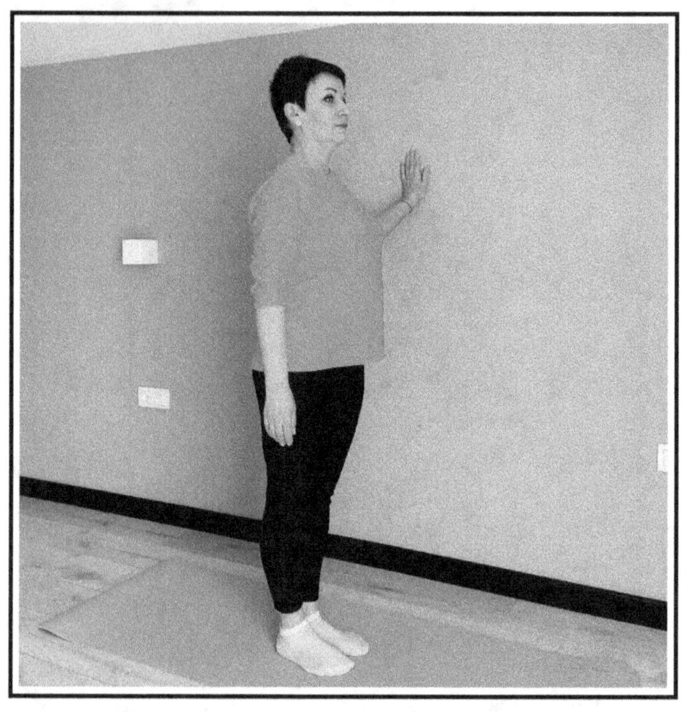

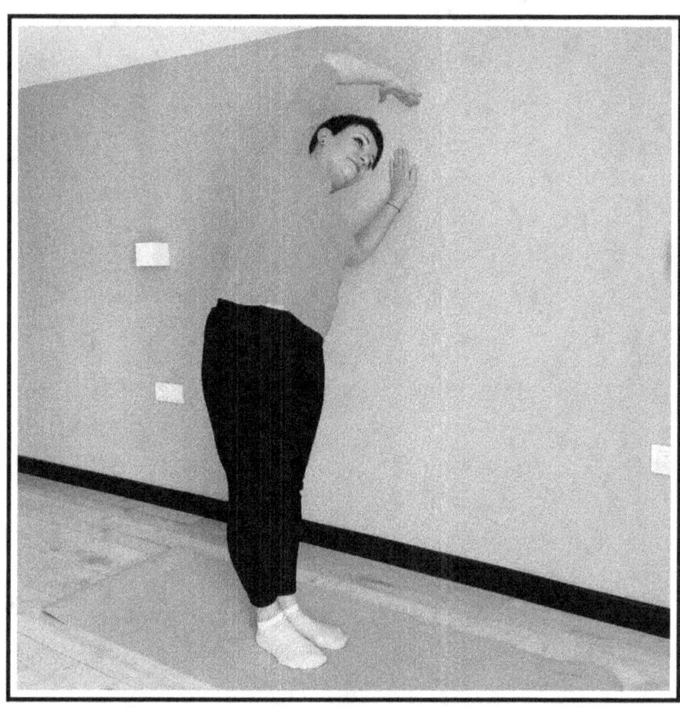

PROCEDURE:

1. Stand with your left side against the wall
2. Place the left hand on the wall
3. Bend toward the left side and, at the same time, lift the right arm up above your head
4. Touch the fingers together; return to the previous position; repeat
5. Perform the same exercise on the opposite side

SUGGESTED TIPS:

- Don't bend the legs
- Don't arch near the lower back
- Try to touch the fingers as close as possible and as far as it is comfortable (it's fine if they don't touch)

Wall-Supported Side Bends

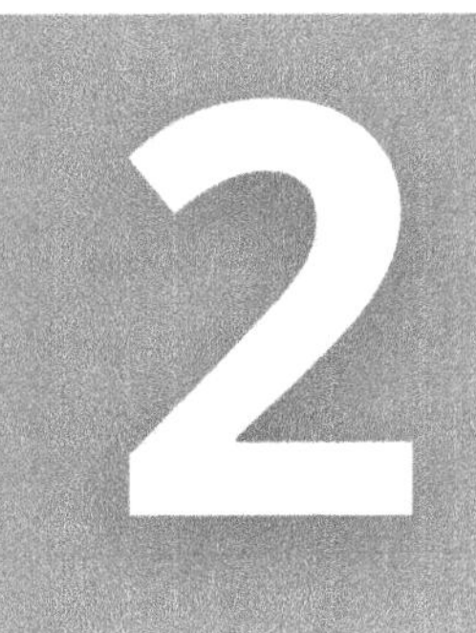

Wall Side Bends are ideal for warming up and stretching your external oblique abdominal muscles and the latissimus dorsi muscle (the large flat muscle in the lower thorax).

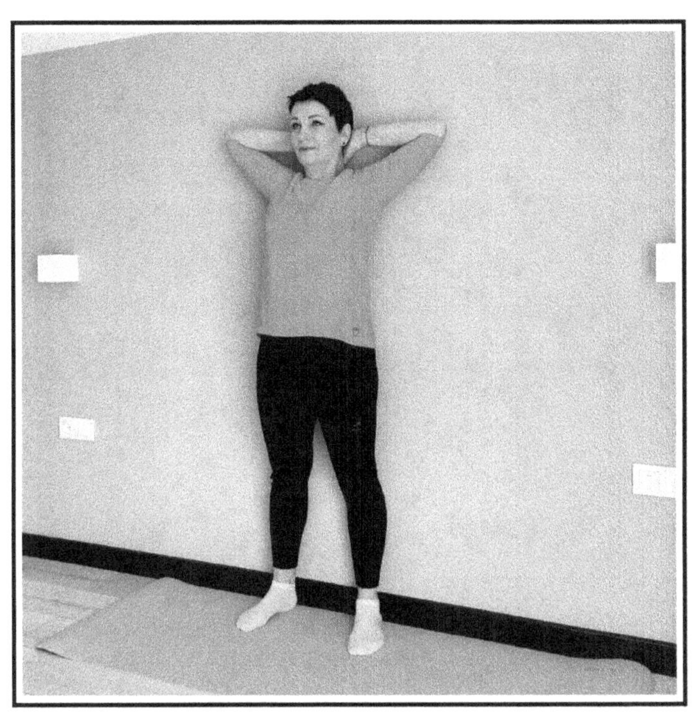 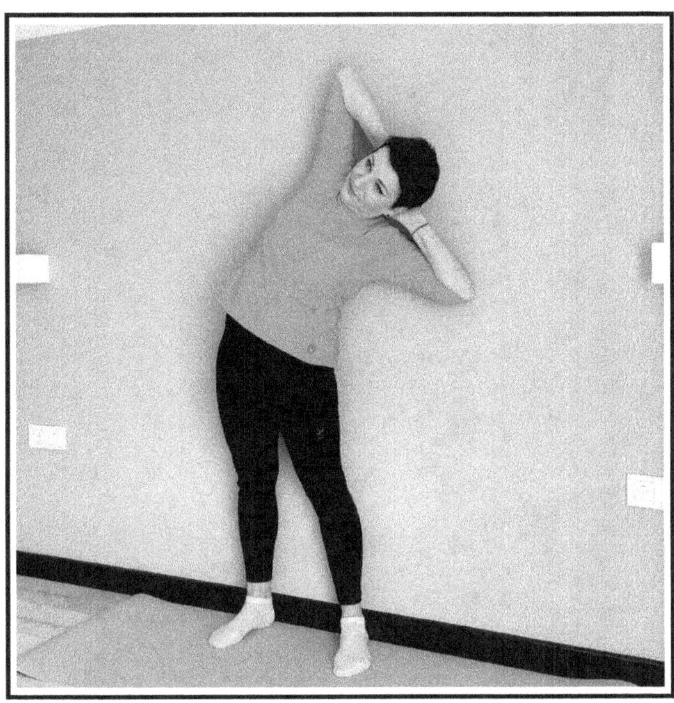

PROCEDURE:

1. Stand tall; have a narrow stance
2. Pin the posterior chain (the muscle groups located on the backside of the body from the upper back to the calf muscles) to the wall
3. Place hands on the backside of the head
4. Bend body sideways; go back up
5. Alternate between sides

SUGGESTED TIPS:

- Don't hold your breath
- Don't move too quickly
- Remember to breathe: inhale at the start of exercise; slowly exhale when bending to the side to engage the stomach muscles

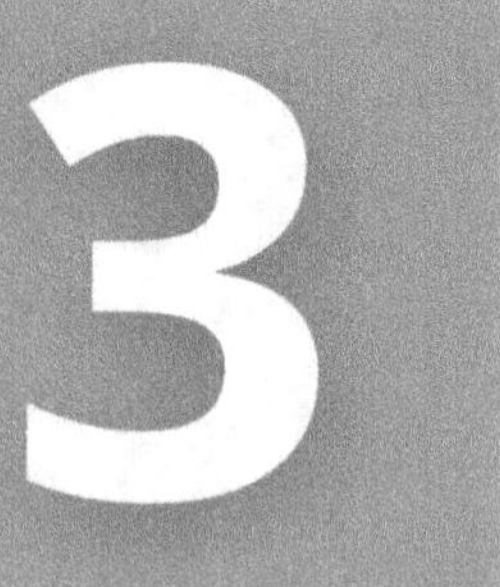

3 Side Leg Swing (Right, Left)

Side Leg Swings help with hip mobility. The exercise is great for a warm-up before doing squats or other lower-body exercises.

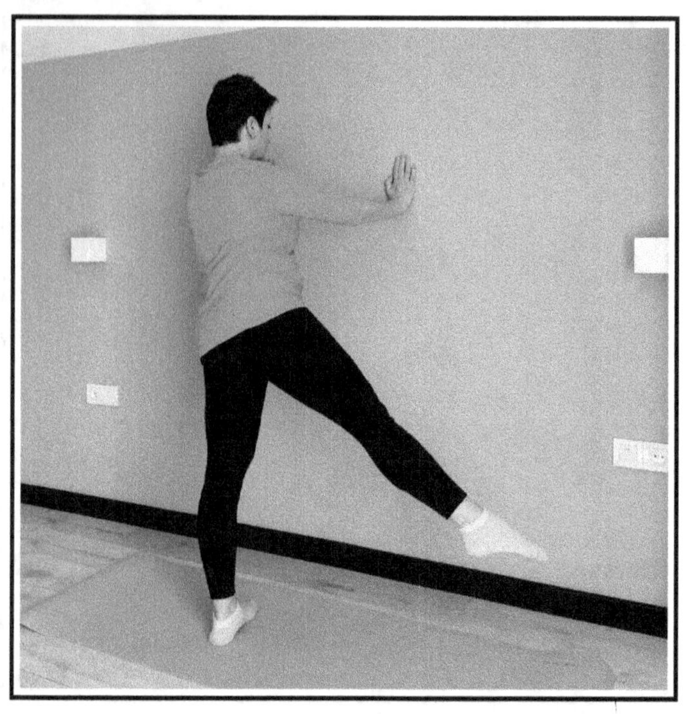

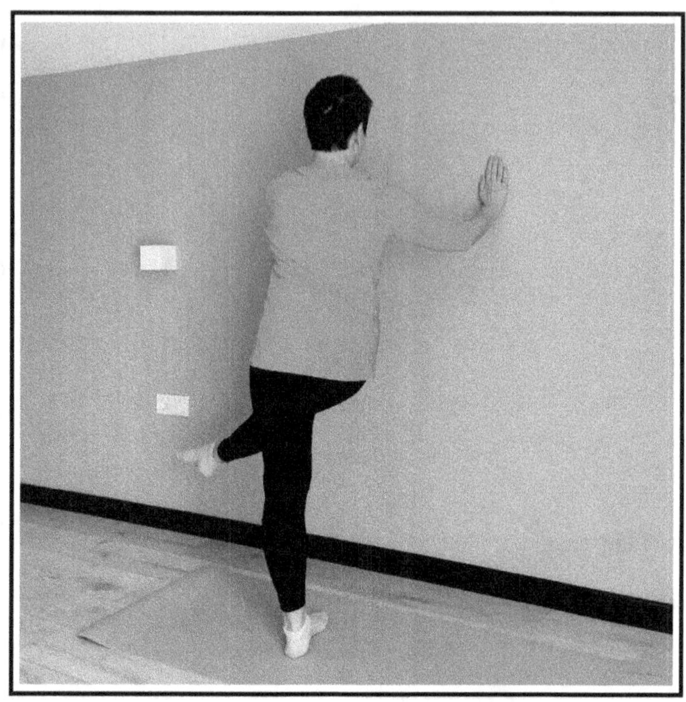

1. Put your feet close together and stand tall
2. Place your hands on the wall
3. Take your right leg and swing to the side, allowing it to come back over your left foot
4. Swing it back again; repeat
5. Perform the same exercise on the opposite side

- Don't bend the knees
- Don't hold your breath
- Continue steady breathing throughout the exercise

Alternating Shoulder Rotations

Alternating Shoulder Rotations are a great exercise to loosen up stiff shoulders and warm them up.

4

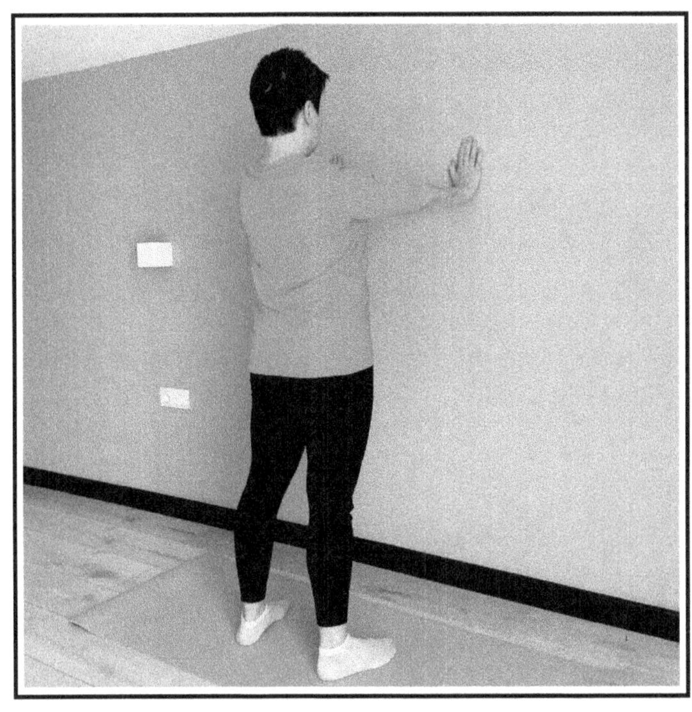
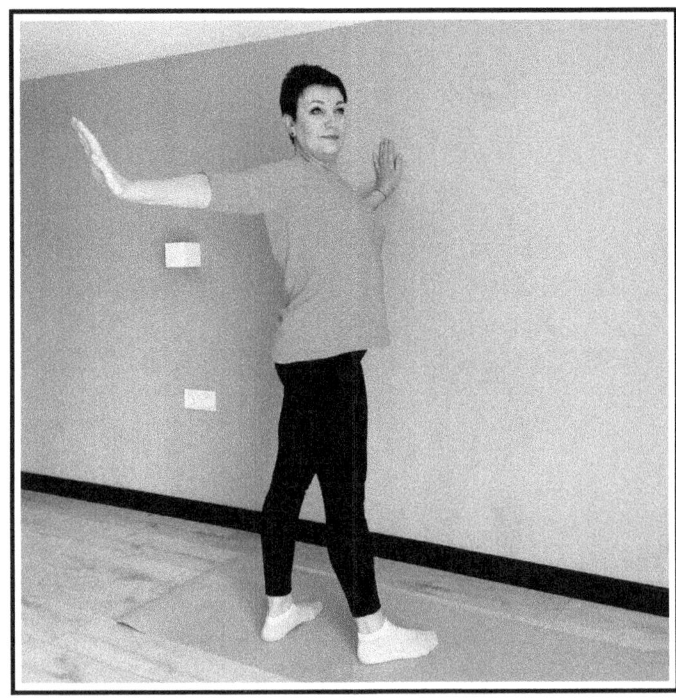

PROCEDURE:

1. Place your feet shoulder-width apart; stand tall
2. Place hands on the wall
3. Lift up and rotate one arm backward
4. Rotate your head gently toward the arm that's rotating
5. Go back up
6. Alternate between sides

SUGGESTED TIPS:

- Don't bend the arms
- Don't do the exercise too quickly
- Throughout the exercise, keep a steady breathing pattern

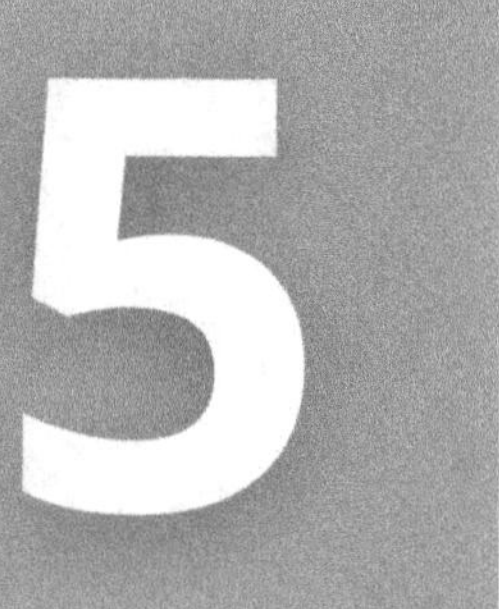

5 Wall Angel

Wall Angles will help reset the posture. They can improve shoulder mobility and activate mid-back muscles.

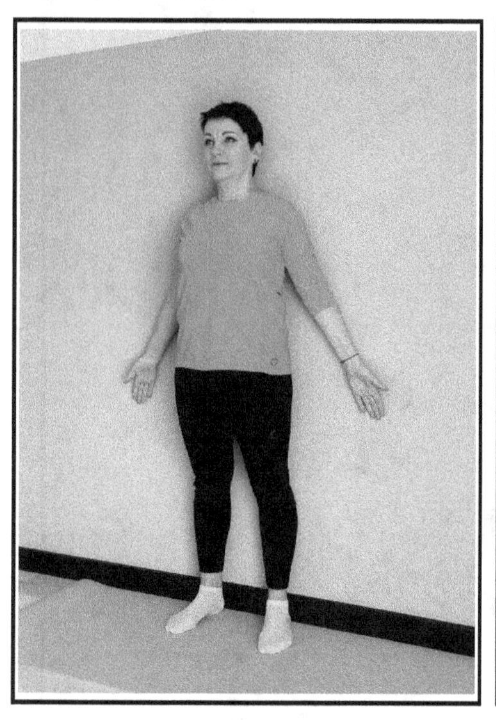
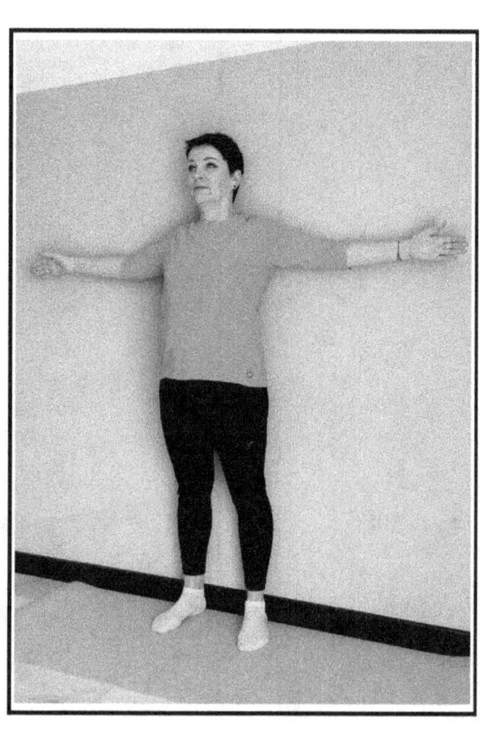
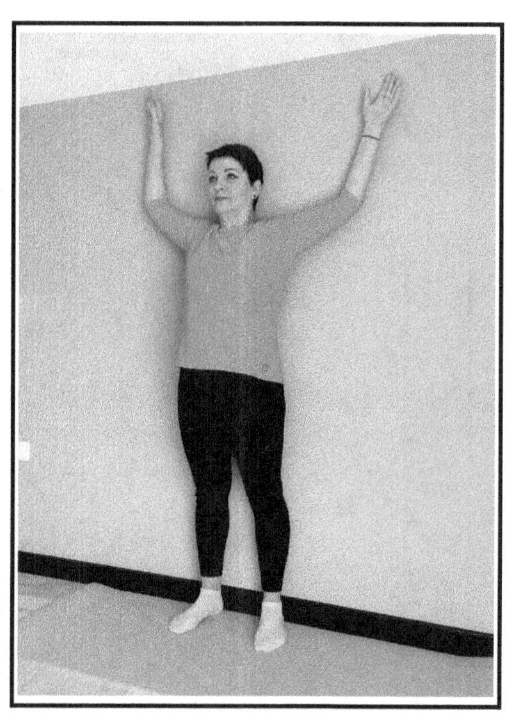

1. Stand tall against the wall
2. Make sure the glutes, back, and head touch the wall
3. Place the hands along the sides
4. Glide the backside all over the wall
5. Slowly go down when the hands touch
6. Repeat the movement

- Don't move too fast
- Don't hold your breath
- Keep your posterior chain against the wall (if this is difficult, take a step forward)

Leg Swing (Right, Left)

Leg Swings improve hip mobility and stretch the hip flexor muscle (using muscles to bring about the stretch, as opposed to traditional "static" stretching).

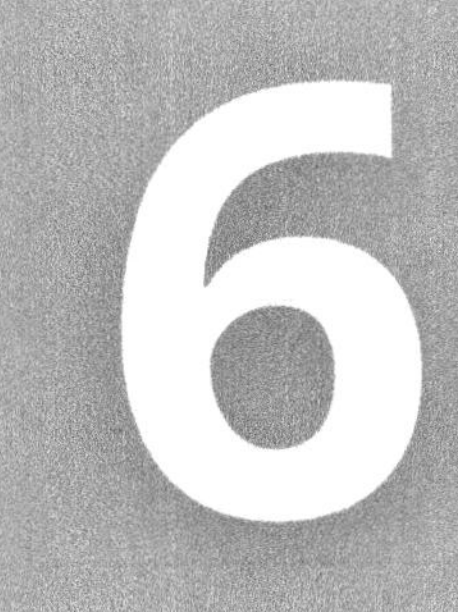

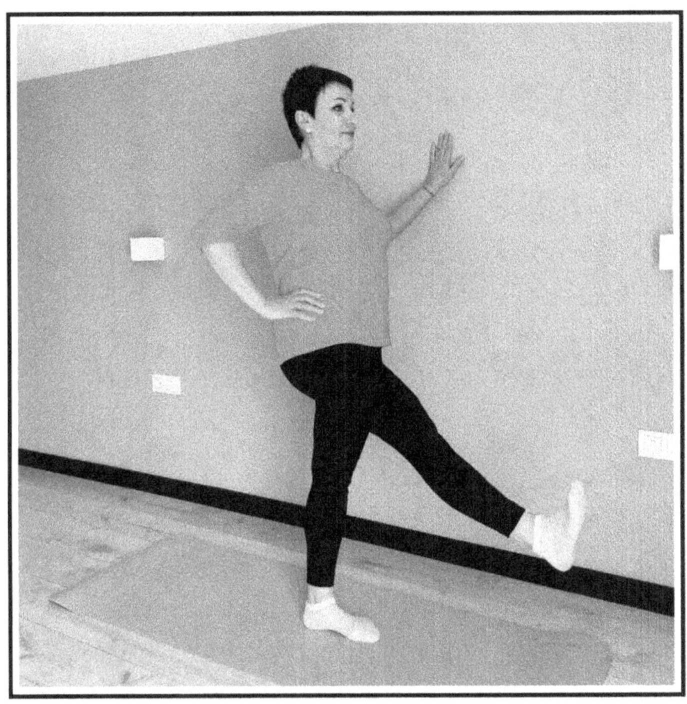

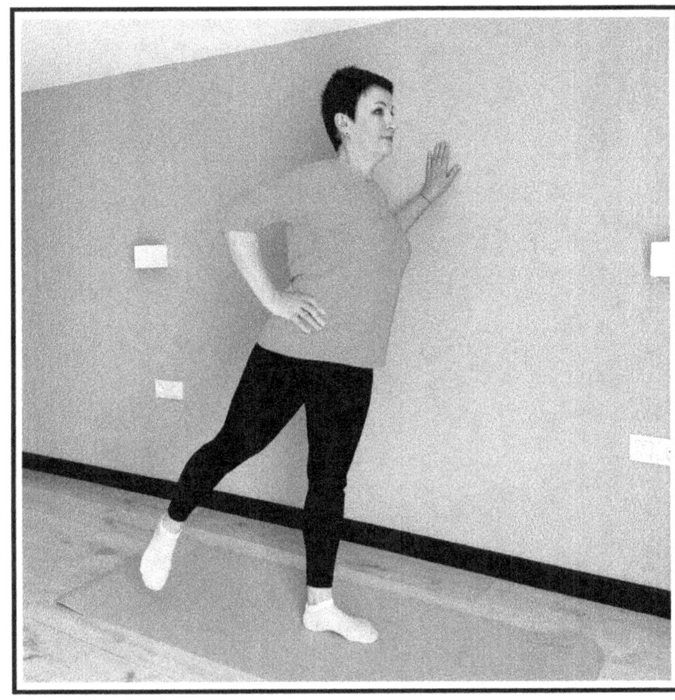

PROCEDURE:

1. Stand with your left side against the wall
2. Place the left hand on the wall
3. Place the right hand on the hip
4. Swing the right leg forward and backward
5. Perform the same exercise with the left leg

SUGGESTED TIPS:

- Don't bend the knees
- Don't hold your breath
- Keep a steady breathing pattern throughout the exercise

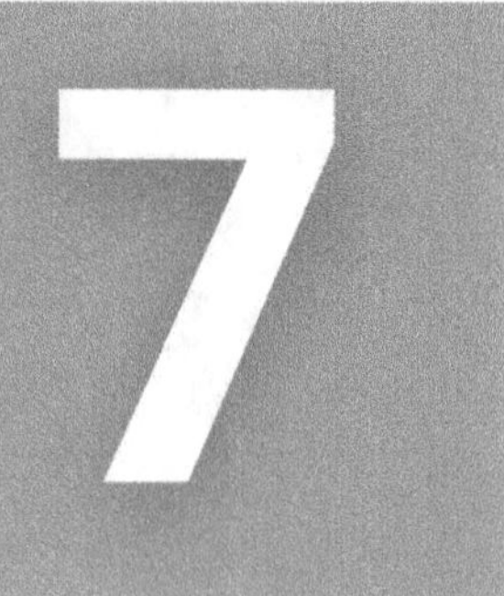

7 Standing Knee Raise
(Right, Left)

Standing Knee Raises help work on stability and activate the hip flexor muscles.

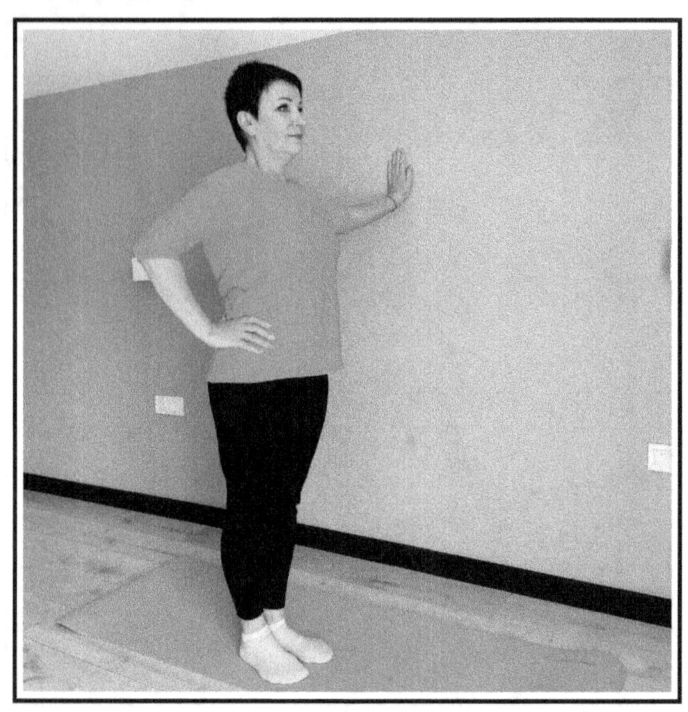 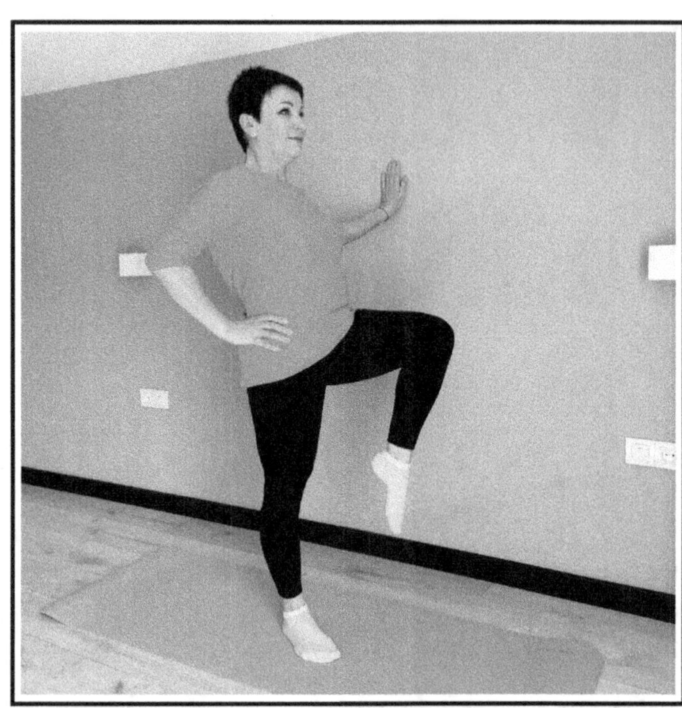

PROCEDURE:

1. Stand with your left side against the wall
2. Place the left hand on the wall
3. Place the right hand on the hip
4. Lift up the left knee
5. Bring the knee down slowly; repeat
6. Turn with your right side against the wall, and perform the same exercise with the right knee

SUGGESTED TIPS:

- Move slowly; take your time
- Don't arch the lower back
- Keep breathing throughout the exercise

Standing Mountain Climbers

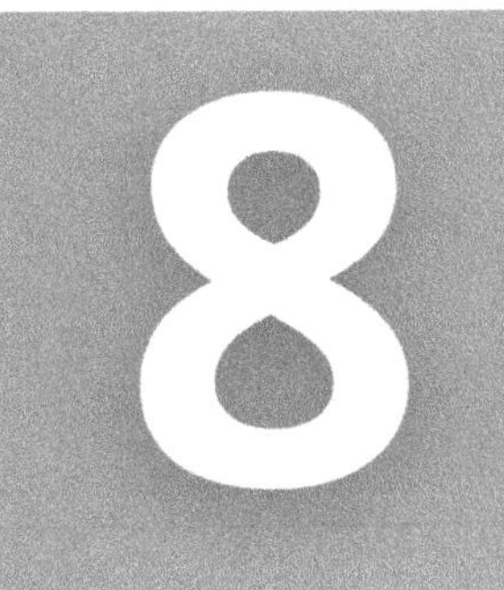

Standing Mountain Climbers improve overall fitness and work the cardiovascular system.

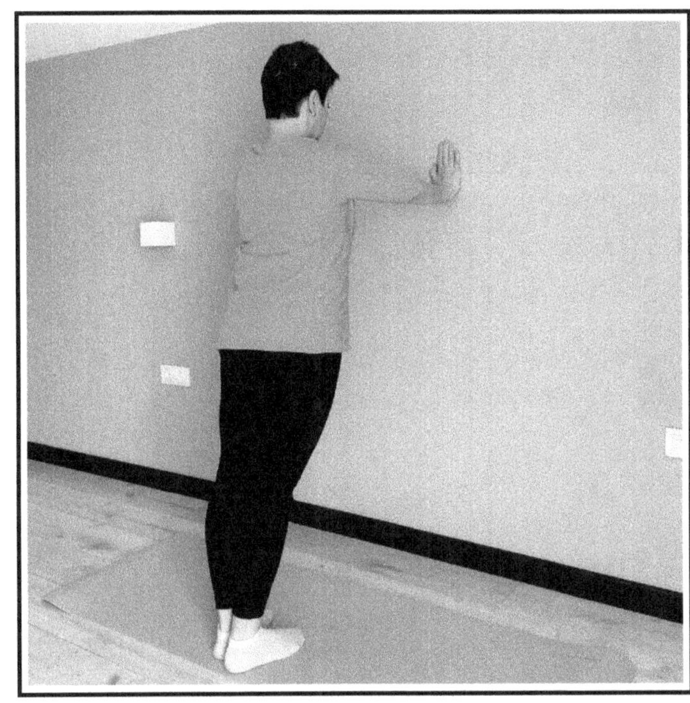

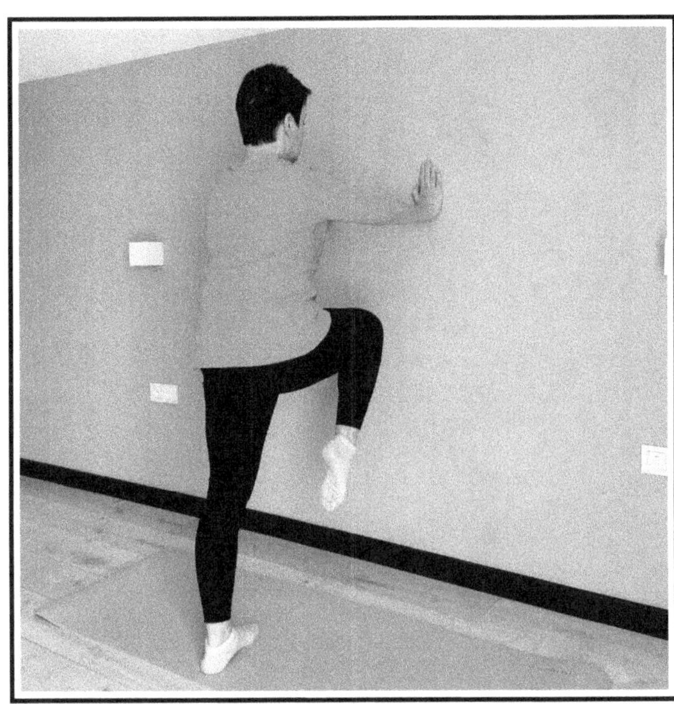

PROCEDURE:

1. Stand tall with feet shoulder-width apart
2. Place the hands on the wall for support
3. Extend the arms
4. Lift up one knee and then put it down; lift up the other knee
5. Repeat the movement

SUGGESTED TIPS:

- Keep the back straight
- Don't hold your breath
- For more challenge, alternate the legs faster

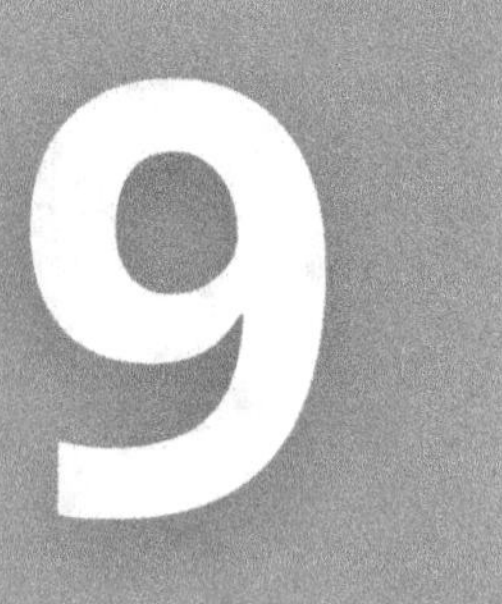

9 Standing Hip Openers

Standing Hip Openers activate the glute muscles and improve hip mobility.

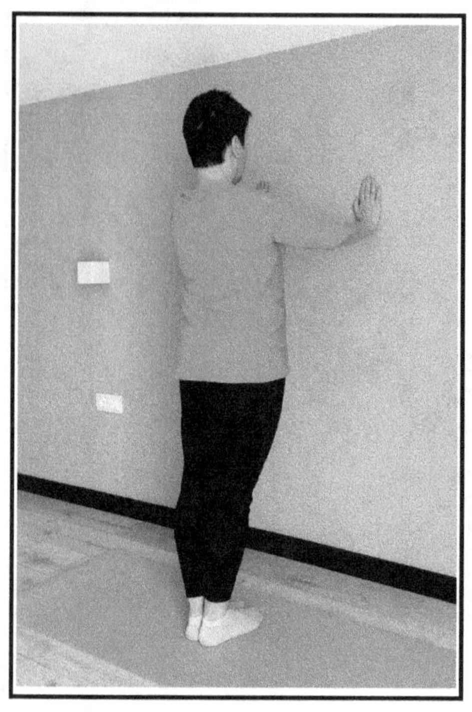 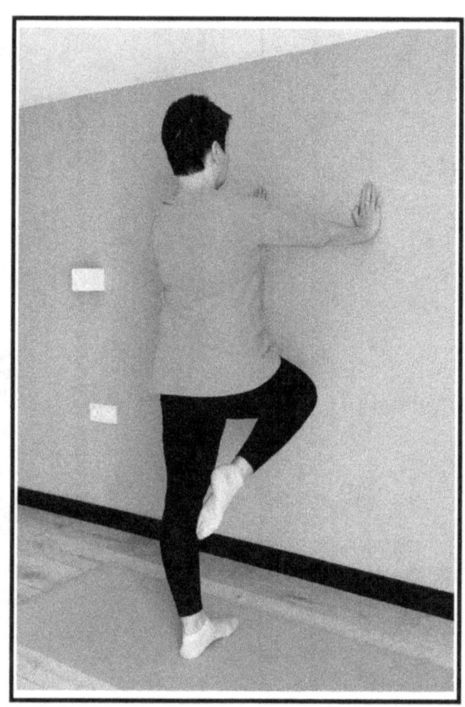 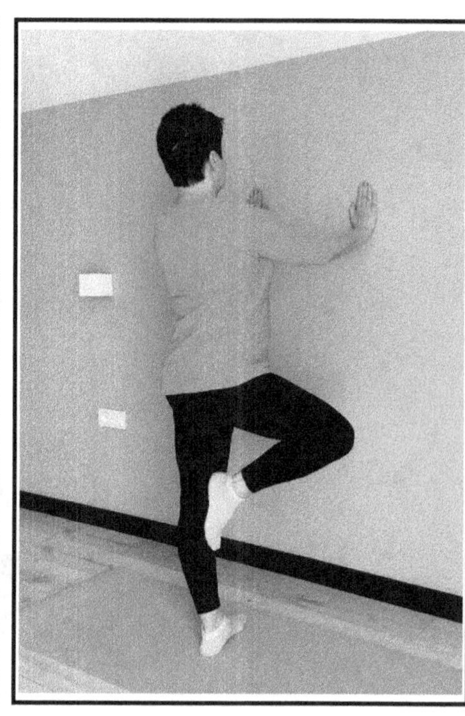

PROCEDURE:

1. With the feet close together, stand as tall as possible
2. Place hands on the wall
3. Slide the right foot over the left leg
4. After reaching as far as possible, open the leg to the side
5. Bring the leg down slowly
6. Alternate between legs

SUGGESTED TIPS:

- Go slowly
- Don't hold your breath
- Keep a steady breathing pattern throughout the exercise

Seated Knee to Chest

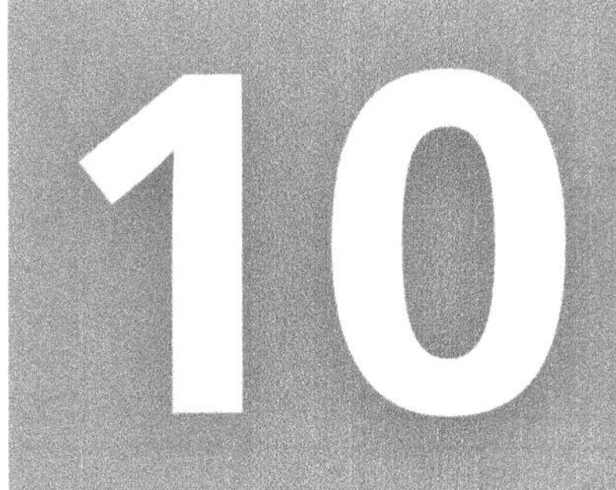

Seated Knee to Chest exercises activate the hip flexor muscles.

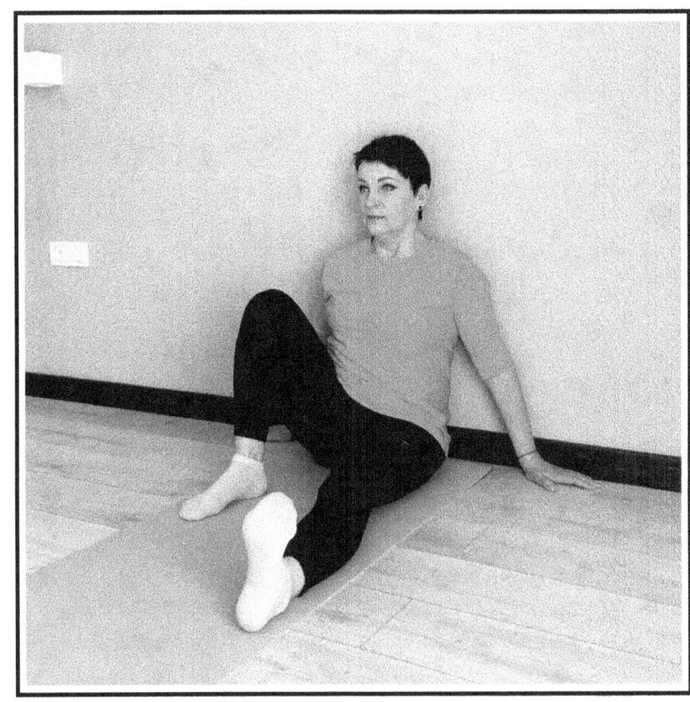 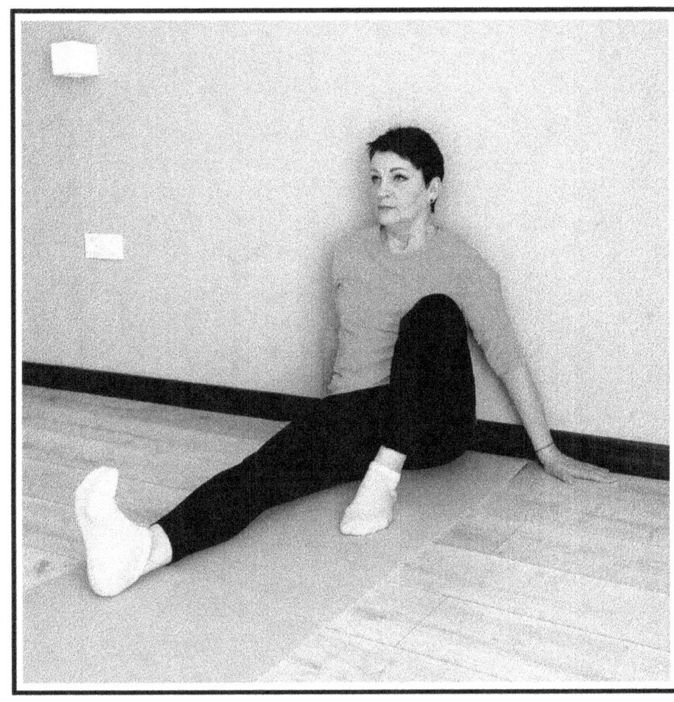

1. Sit up tall against the wall
2. Place the hands to the sides
3. Extend the legs
4. Slide a knee to the chest without lifting the leg; bring back
5. Alternate between legs

- Don't arch the lower back
- Keep a steady breathing pattern throughout the exercise

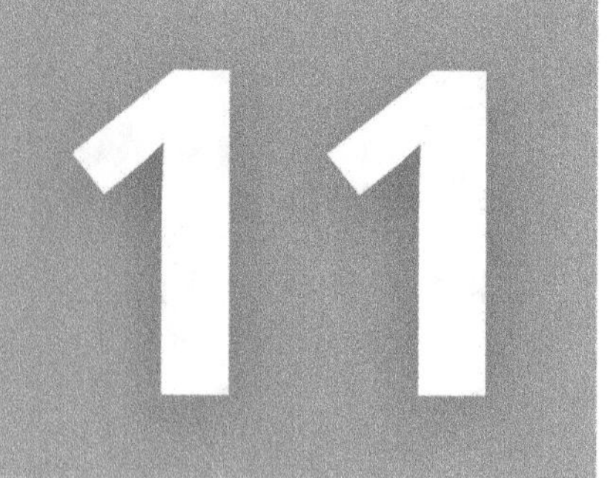

Supported Spine Twist

Supported Spine Twist exercises increase thoracic spine mobility which, in turn, improves shoulder movement. Feeling some mid-back tightness... then this exercise is a perfect fit!

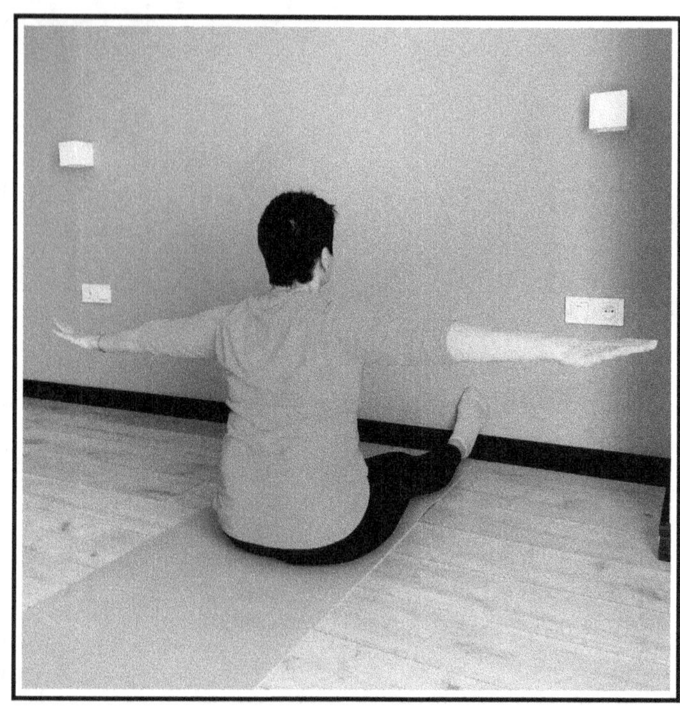 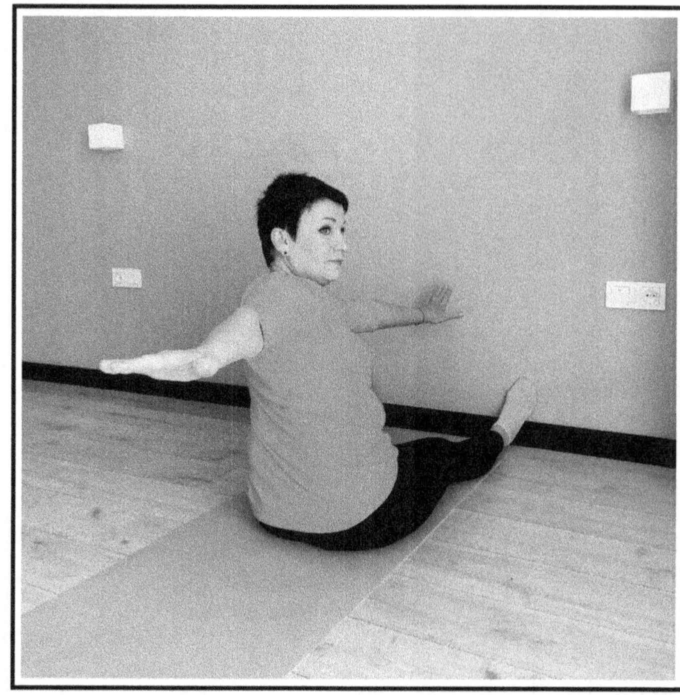

1. Sit up tall while facing the wall
2. Straddle the legs; place your feet on the wall
3. Extend the arms by the sides
4. Now rotate the torso and head toward one side; bring back
5. Alternate between sides

- Don't bend the knees
- Don't bend the back
- Take your time; move slowly
- At the beginning of the exercise, inhale; as you rotate the torso, slowly exhale

Exercises for Legs and Glutes

Alternating Side Hip Slides

Alternating Side Hip Slides help work the pectoralis muscle (the largest muscle of the anterior chest wall) and strengthen the adductor muscles of the hip used mostly to bring the thighs together. This exercise helps with external hip mobility.

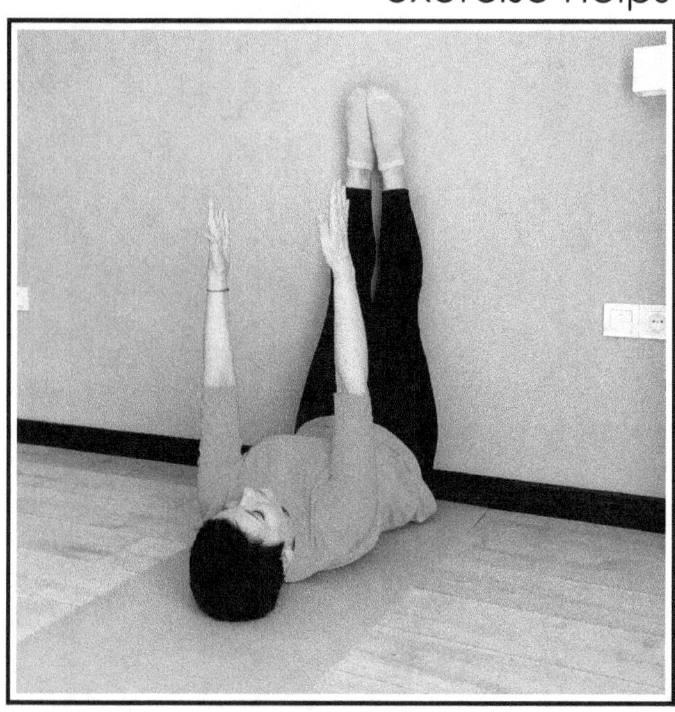
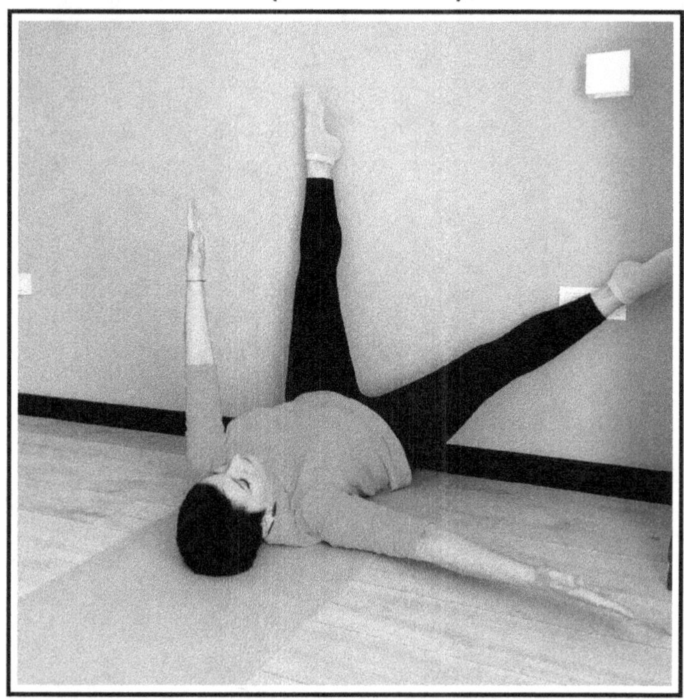

PROCEDURE:

1. Lay down on your back
2. Extend the legs on the wall
3. Extend the arms out
4. At the same time, bring the right arm and right leg down
5. Go back up
6. Alternate between arms and legs

SUGGESTED TIPS:

- Don't move the pelvis around (imagine pushing the bellybutton to the floor)
- Don't arch the lower back
- Remember to breathe

Butterfly Openers

Butterfly Openers activate the pectoral muscles (the muscles that connect the front of the chest with the bones of the upper arm and shoulder) and work the external hip rotation.

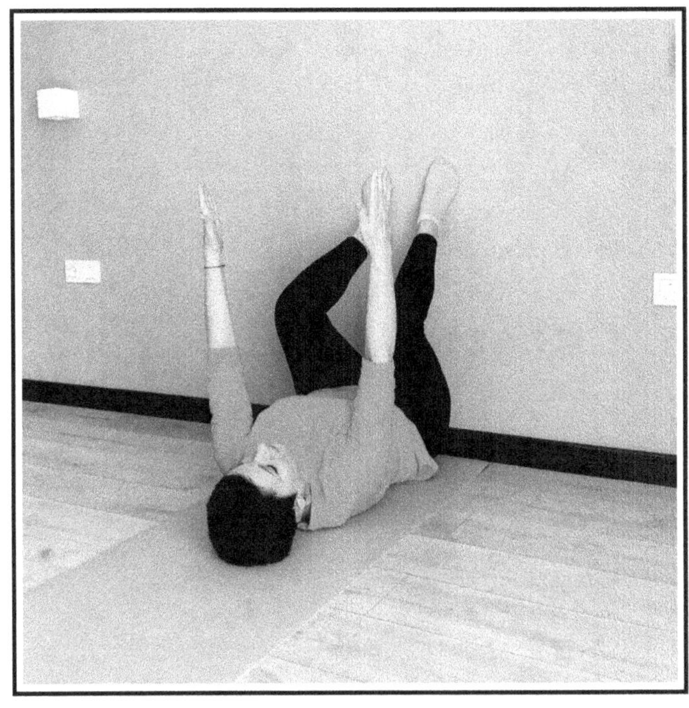

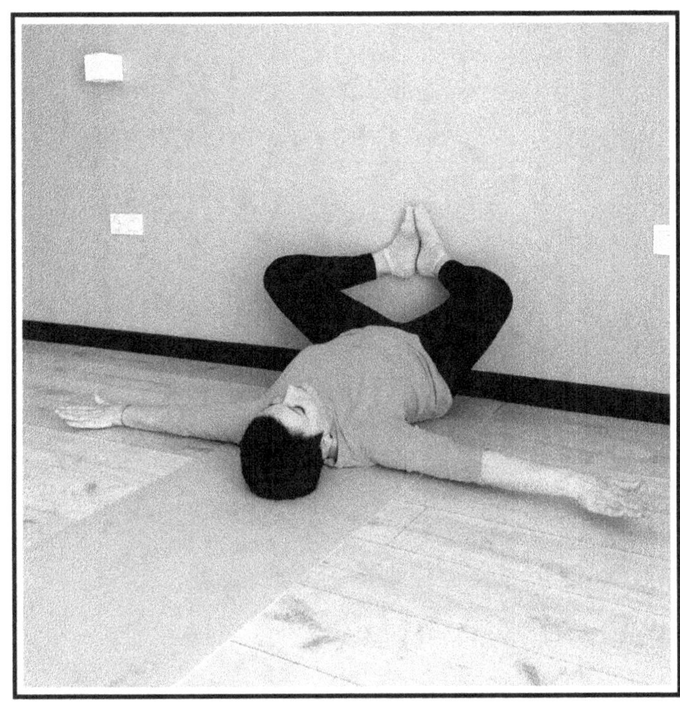

PROCEDURE:

1. Lay down on your back
2. Extend the arms out
3. Keep the feet on the wall
4. Bend the knees at a 90-degree angle
5. At the same time, open the arms and knees
6. Then bring them back
7. Repeat the movement

SUGGESTED TIPS:

- Take your time
- Don't arch the back
- Continue to breathe throughout the exercise
- At the beginning of the exercise, inhale; as you open the arms and legs, slowly exhale

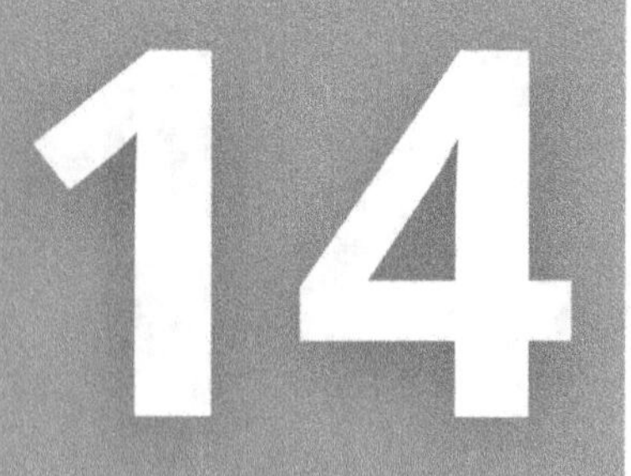

14 Knee to Chest (Right, Left)

Knee to Chest exercises build hip flexor strength and activate the hip flexor muscle.

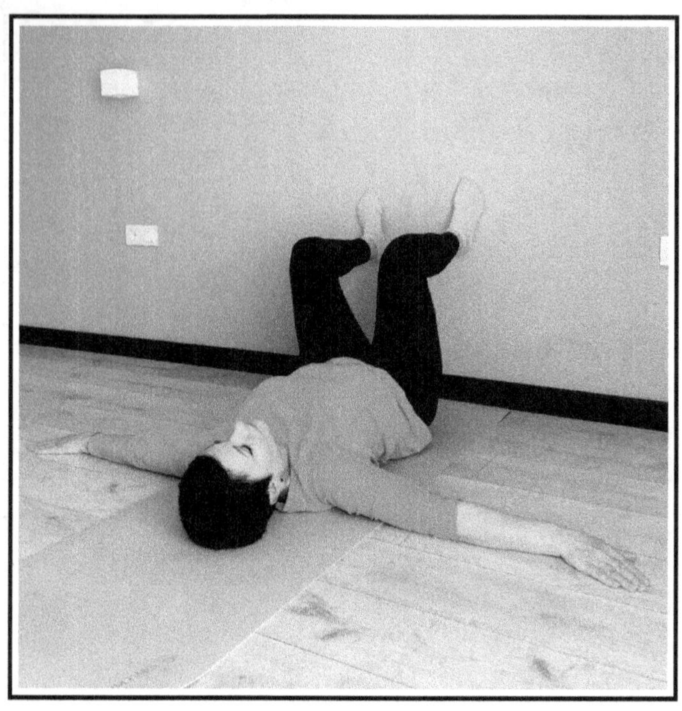 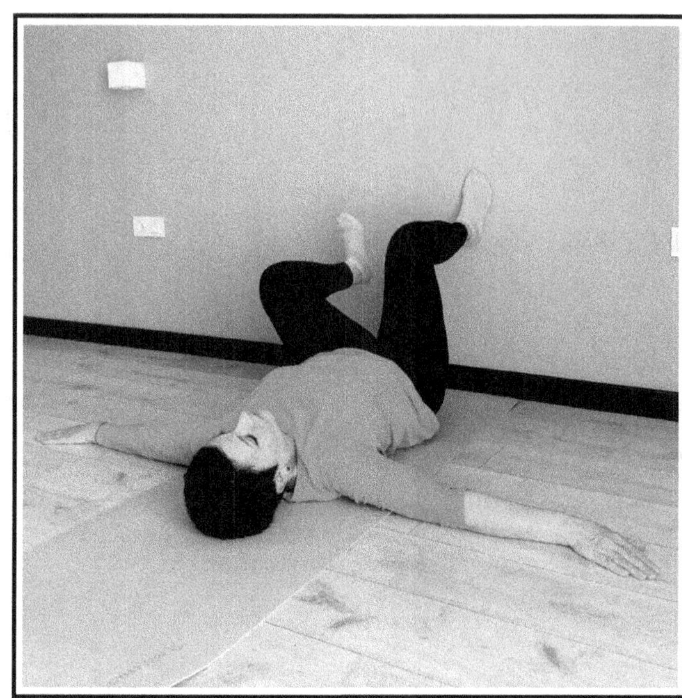

PROCEDURE:

1. Lay down on your back
2. Bend the knees at a 90-degree angle on the wall
3. Extend arms to the sides
4. Lift up the left knee and bring it to the chest
5. Go back up; repeat the exercise
6. Perform the same exercise with the right knee

SUGGESTED TIPS:

- Take your time
- Continue to breathe throughout the exercise (maintain a steady breathing pattern)
- Don't arch the back

PAGE 32

Unilateral Wall Slides

Unilateral Wall Slides activate the hip flexors and the hamstring muscles.

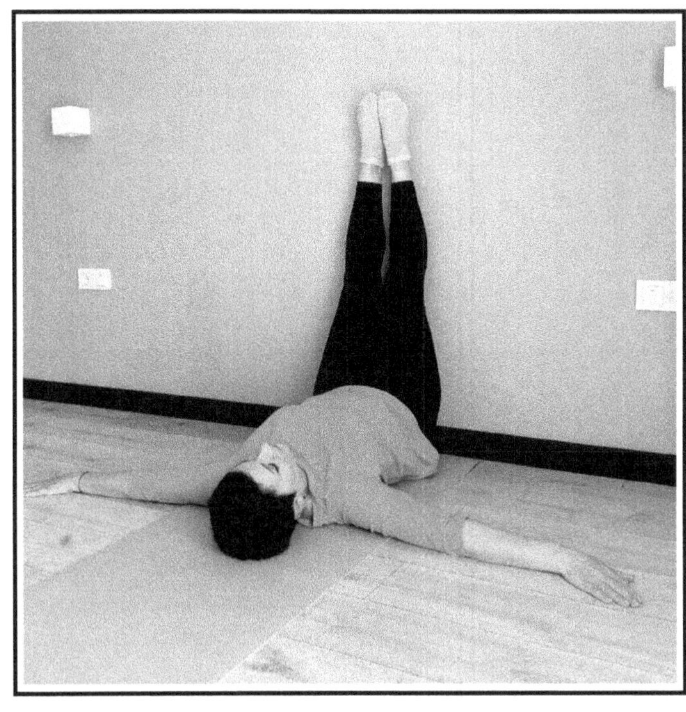 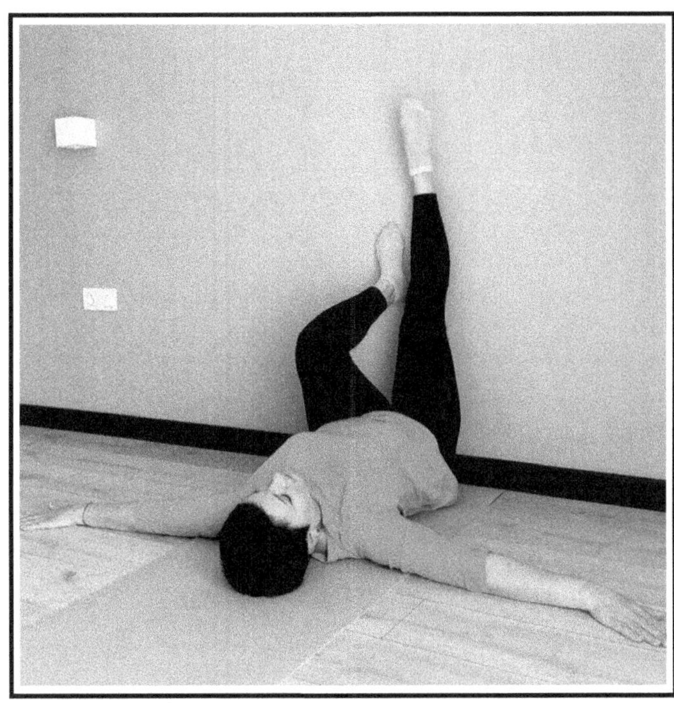

1. Lay down on your back
2. Extend the knees on the wall
3. Keep heels on the wall
4. Slide left foot down; extend back up
5. Alternate between arms and legs

- Don't arch the lower back
- Continue breathing throughout the exercise
- At the beginning of the exercise, inhale; as you slide the foot down, exhale

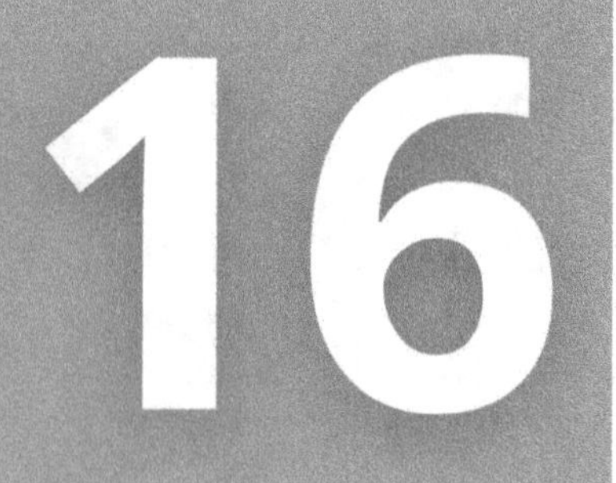

16 Wall Hip Opener

Wall Hip Openers activate the hamstring muscles and work the external hip rotation.

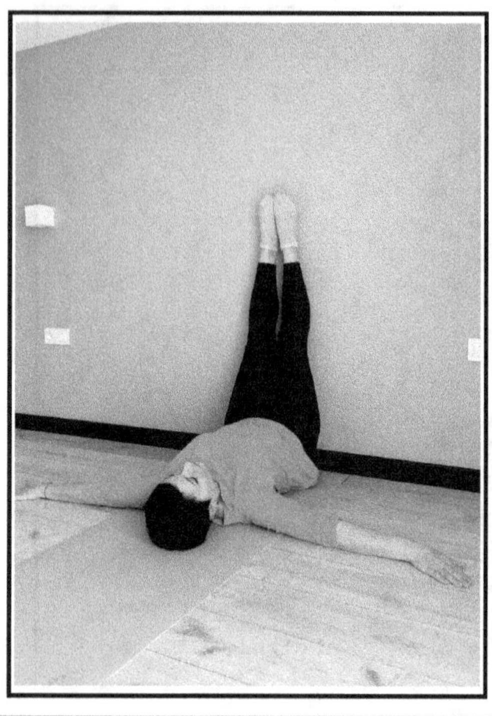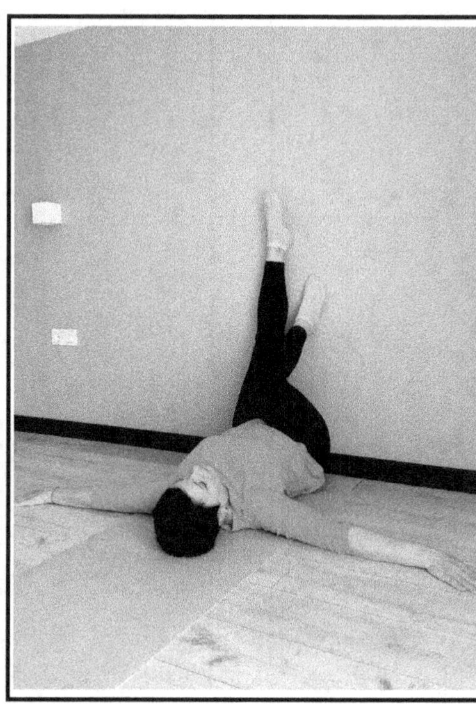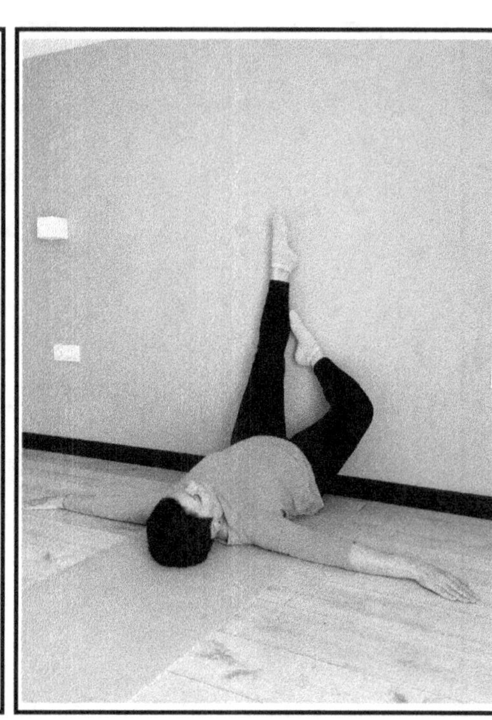

PROCEDURE:

1. Lay down on your back
2. Extend knees on the wall
3. Keep heels on the wall
4. Slide right foot down; open knee to side
5. Bring it inward; slide it back up
6. Alternate between legs

SUGGESTED TIPS:

- Don't arch the lower back
- Continue breathing throughout the exercise (maintain a steady breathing pattern)

Zig-Zag

Zig-Zags are an ideal exercise if your hips are tight. They work out internal and external hip mobility.

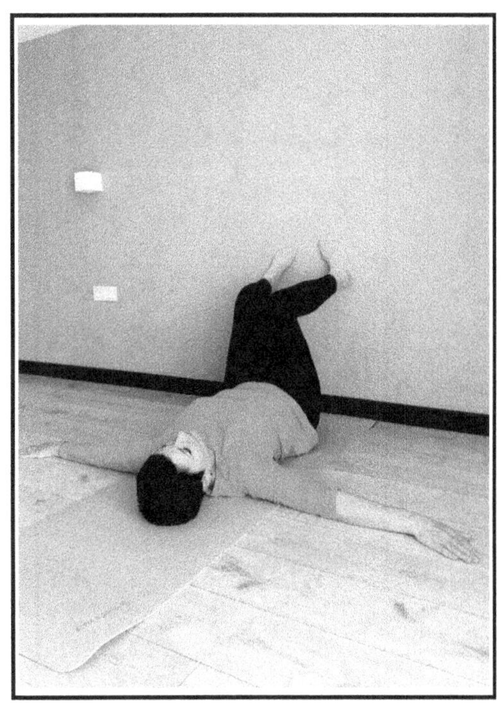 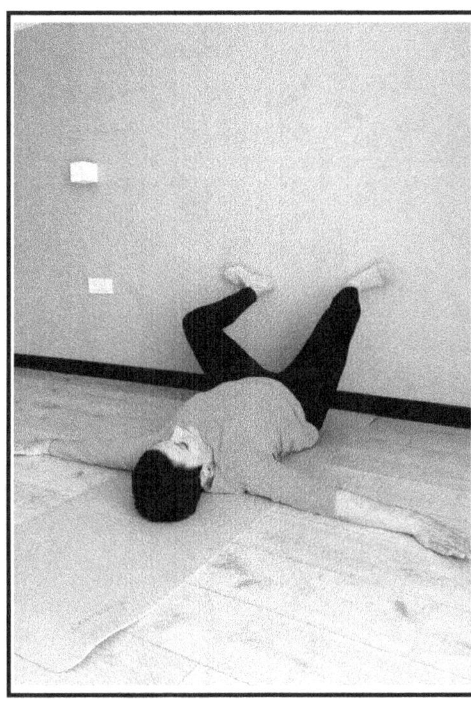 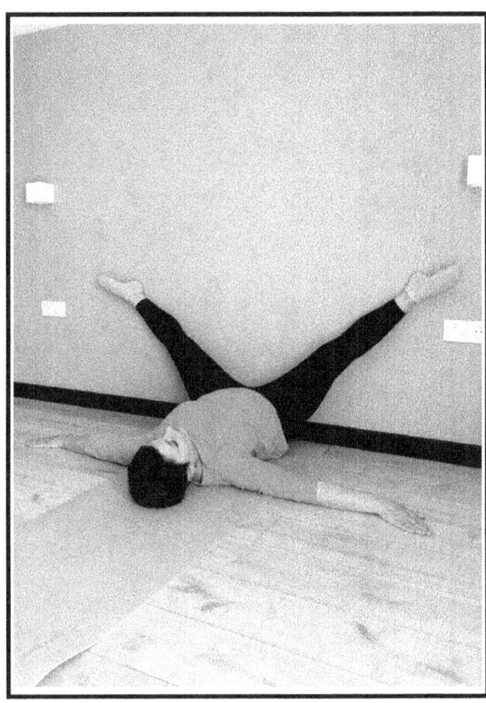

PROCEDURE:

1. Lay down on your back
2. Place the feet at a 90-degree angle on the wall
3. Rotate the knees inward to touch each other
4. Open the knees to the side
5. Slide the feet up
6. As you rotate the knees inward, bring the feet down
7. Repeat the movement

SUGGESTED TIPS:

- Don't arch the lower back
- Take your time
- Continue to breathe throughout the exercise (maintain a steady breathing pattern)

18 Alternating Leg Abduction

The Alternating Leg Abduction exercises stretch the adductor muscles and work on hip mobility.

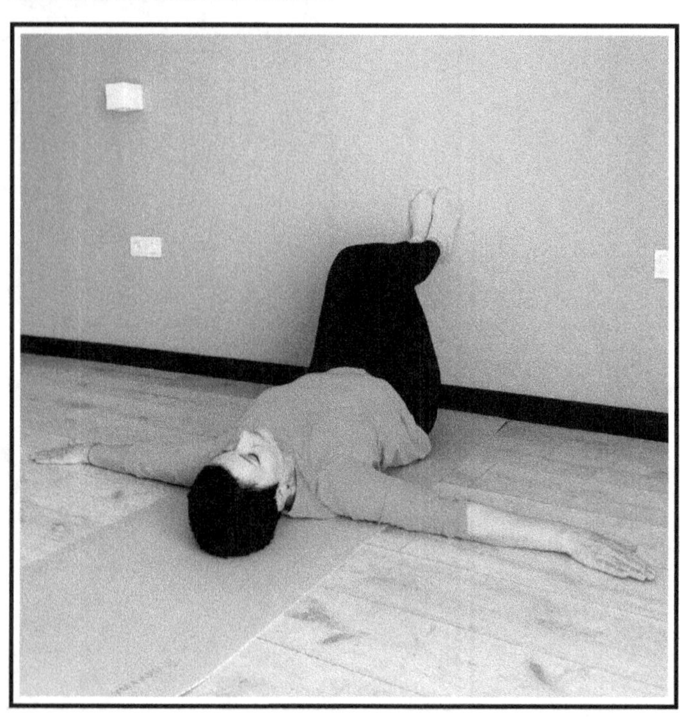 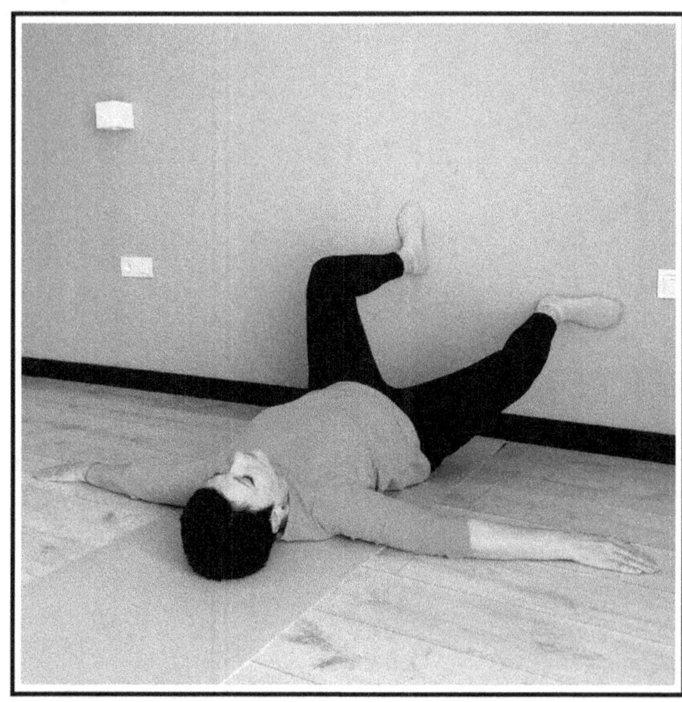

PROCEDURE:

1. Lay down on your back
2. Extend arms out to the sides
3. Place the feet on the wall with knees at 90 degrees
4. Slide a foot down to the side; bring it back
5. Alternate between legs

SUGGESTED TIPS:

- Don't arch the lower back
- Keep the pelvis on the floor (imagine pushing the bellybutton to the floor)

Double Knee Bends

The Double Knee Bends activate the hip flexors and hamstrings. The exercise stretches the latissimus dorsi muscle (the large flat muscle in the thorax).

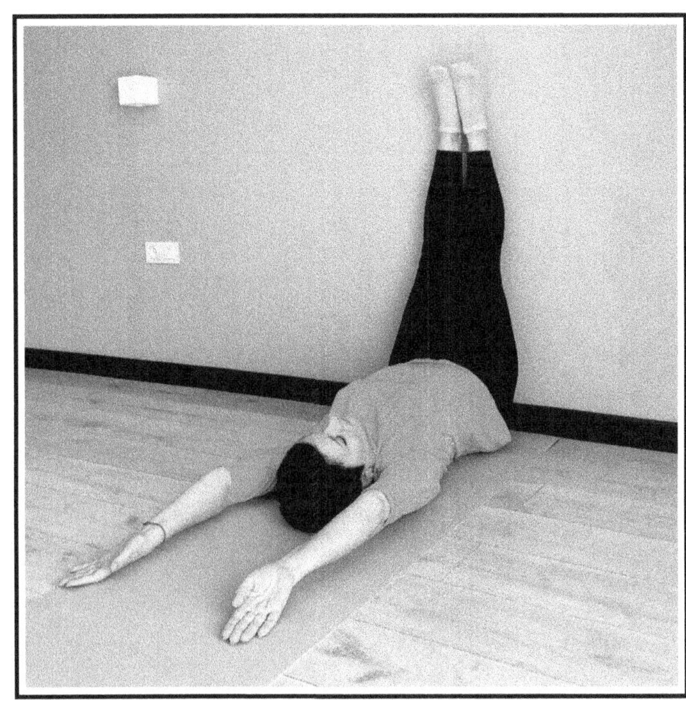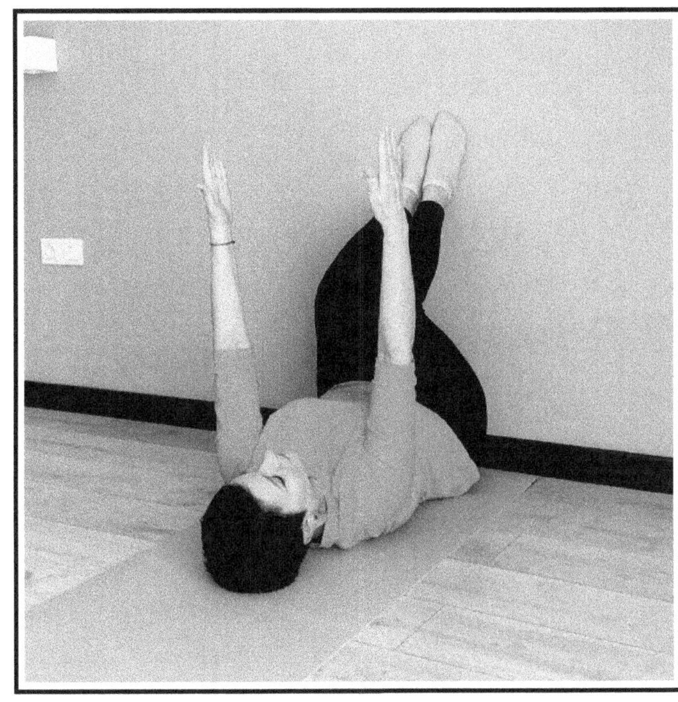

PROCEDURE:

1. Lay down on your back
2. Extend the knees on the wall
3. Engage the abdominals
4. Extend the arms by your head
5. Slide the feet down and bring the elbows toward the knees
6. Go back down
7. Repeat the movement

SUGGESTED TIPS:

- Take your time
- Don't arch the back
- Remember to engage the abdominals
- At the beginning of the exercise, inhale; as you start to bring your arms down, exhale

20 Lying Down Walks

Lying Down Walks exercises will activate the hamstring and glute muscles.

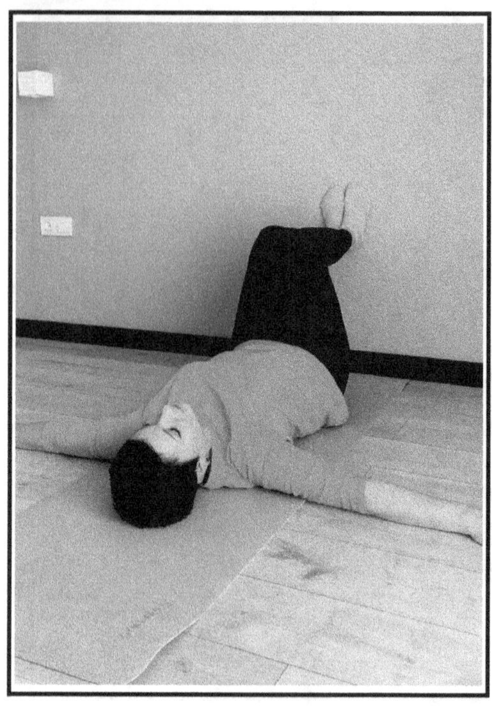 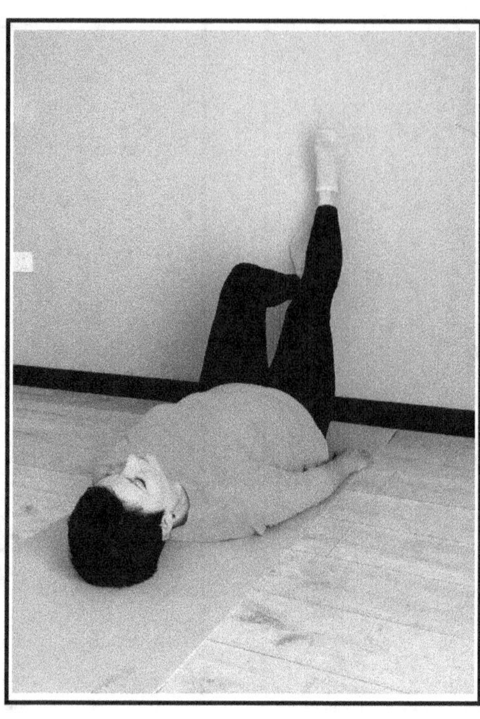 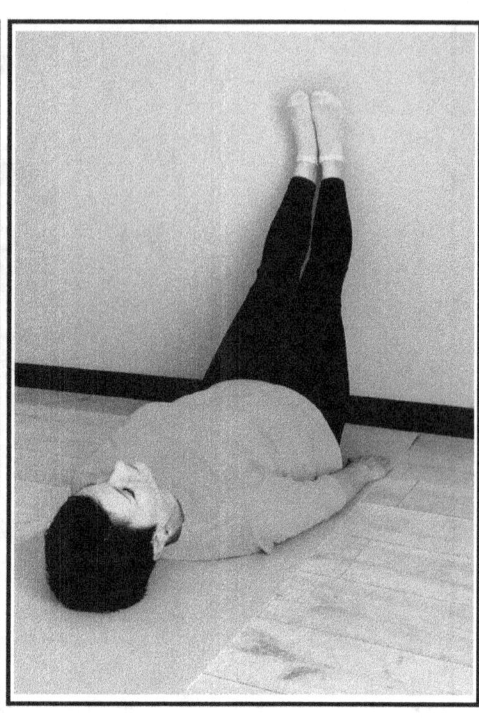

PROCEDURE:

1. Lay down on your back
2. Place the knees on the wall at a 90-degree angle
3. Extend a leg up, then the other one
4. Bring one leg down, then the other one; pretend to walk

SUGGESTED TIPS:

- Don't hold your breath
- Don't arch the lower back
- Continue breathing throughout the exercise (maintain a steady breathing pattern)

Wall Glute Bridge

Wall Glute Bridges are a perfect exercise to fire up the hamstring muscles and the glute.

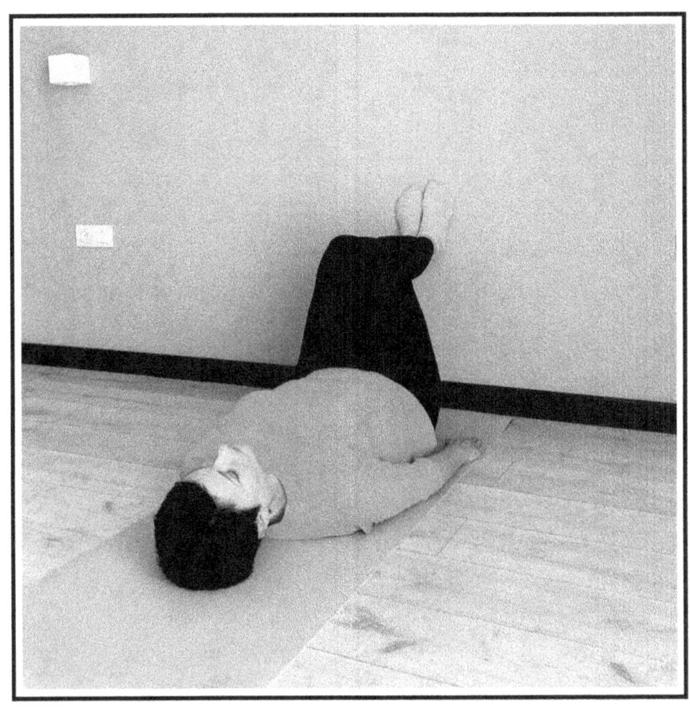 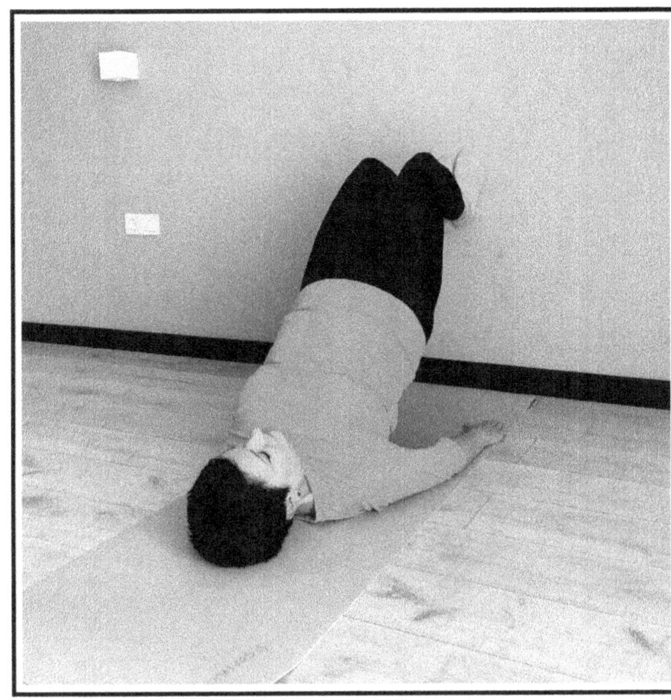

PROCEDURE:

1. Lay down on your back
2. Keep both hands near the sides
3. Put your feet at 90 degrees on the wall
4. Tighten the glute and abdominal muscles
5. Lift the hips up
6. Move slowly as you go down
7. Repeat the exercise

SUGGESTED TIPS:

- Don't arch the lower back
- Make sure to go high enough
- Lower the body slowly; don't drop yourself down. To increase the hamstring activation, drive the heels down when you lift up the hips

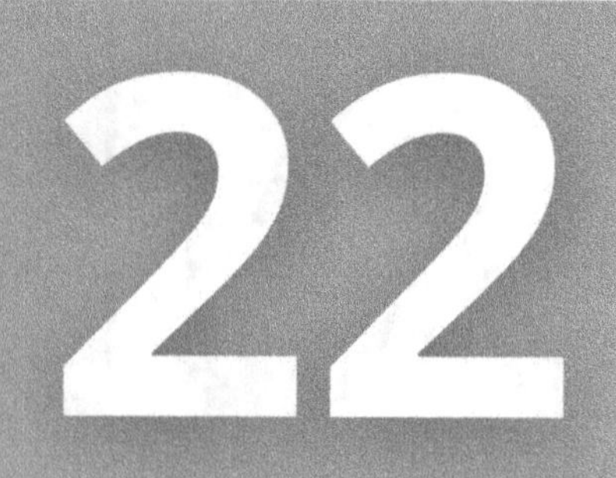

22 Lying Down Walks to Bridge

Lying Down Walks to Bridge exercises will activate the hamstring and glute muscles.

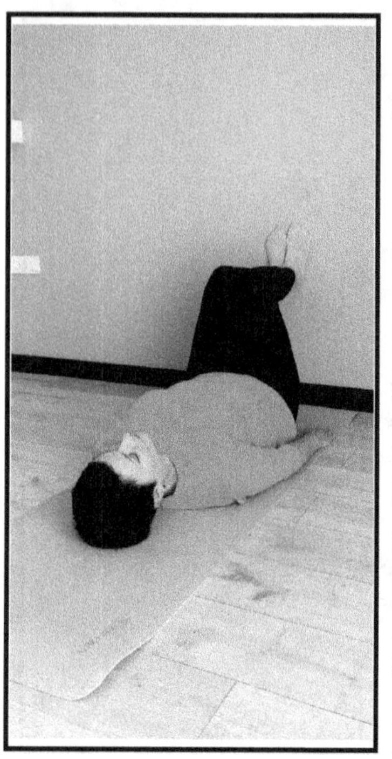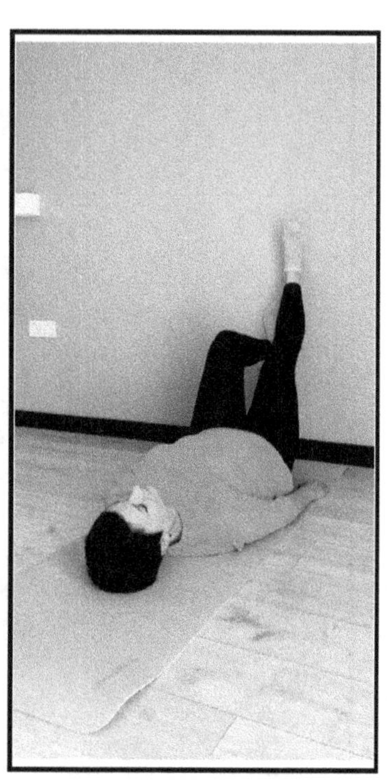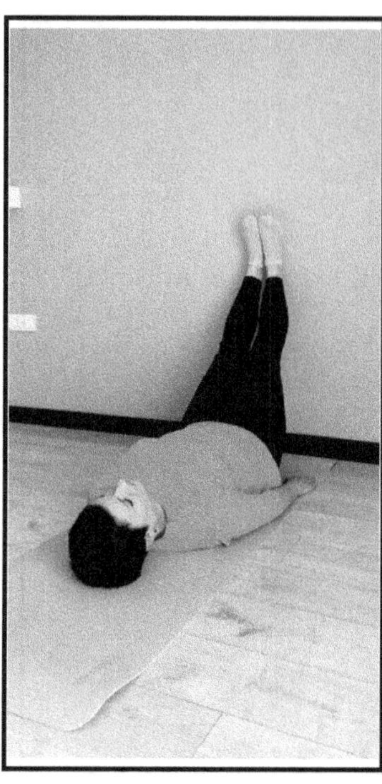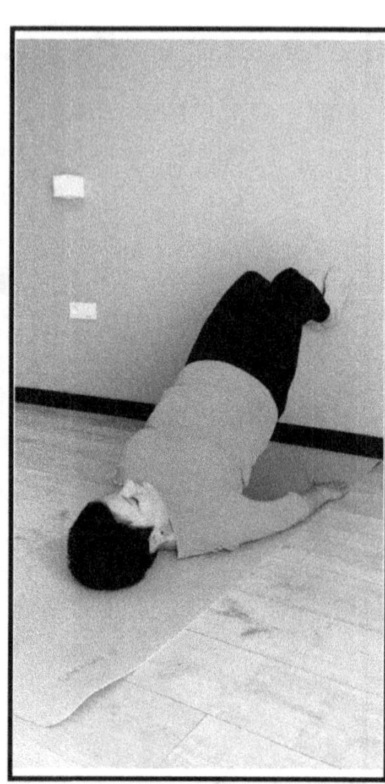

PROCEDURE:

1. Lay down on your back
2. Place the knees on the wall at a 90-degree angle
3. Extend a leg up, then the other one
4. Bend the knees to the starting position; push the hips up
5. Go down; repeat the movement

SUGGESTED TIPS:

- Don't hold your breath
- Don't arch the lower back
- Lower the hips down with control

Lifted Knee to Chest
(Right, Left)

This exercise fires up the hamstring muscles and the glutes (the large muscles on the buttocks). It is a difficult variation of a bridge exercise.

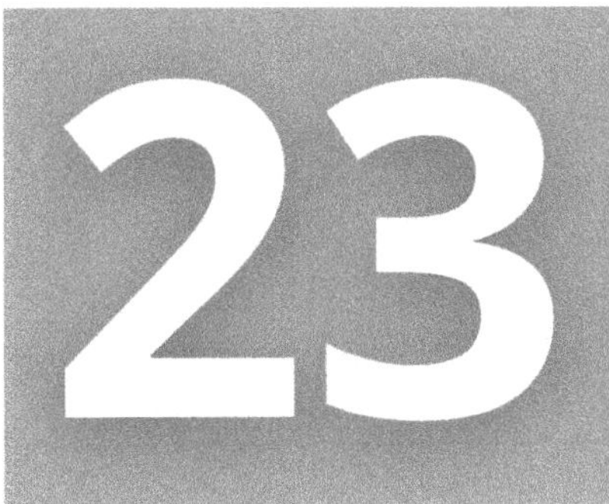

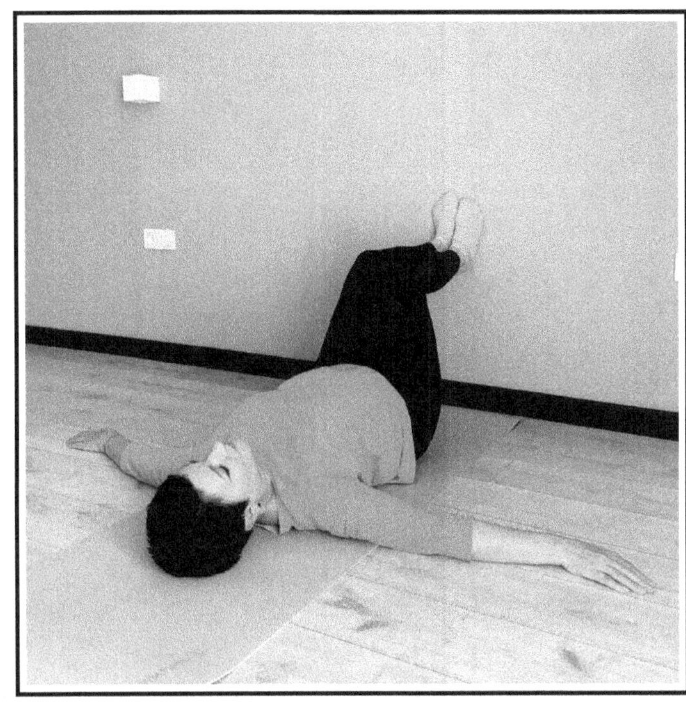

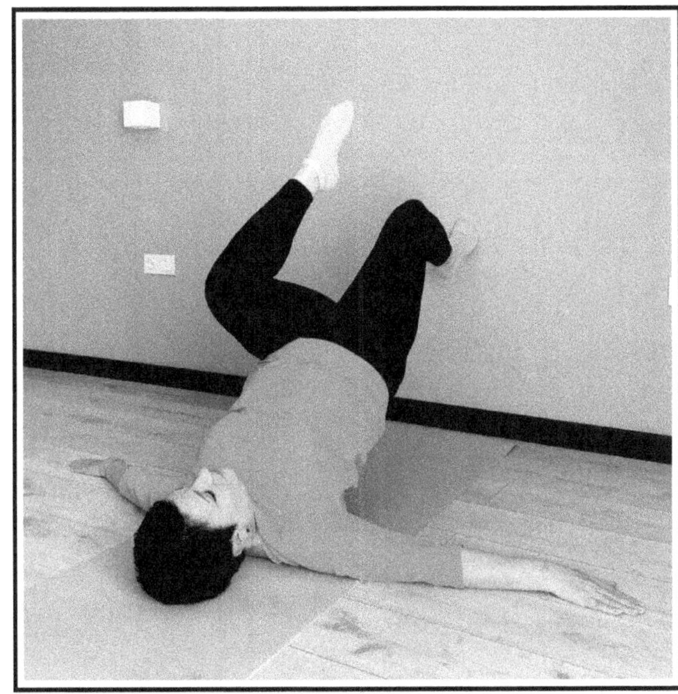

PROCEDURE:

1. Lay down on your back
2. Place the knees on the wall at a 90-degree angle
3. Extend the arms out to the sides
4. With your right foot, push off the wall; bring your hips up
5. At the same time, bring the left knee toward your chest;
6. Go back up; repeat the exercise
7. Perform the same exercise with the other foot and knee

SUGGESTED TIPS:

- Don't go too fast
- Don't arch the lower back (gently contracting the abdominal muscles will help prevent the arching)
- Continue breathing throughout the exercise (maintain a steady breathing pattern)

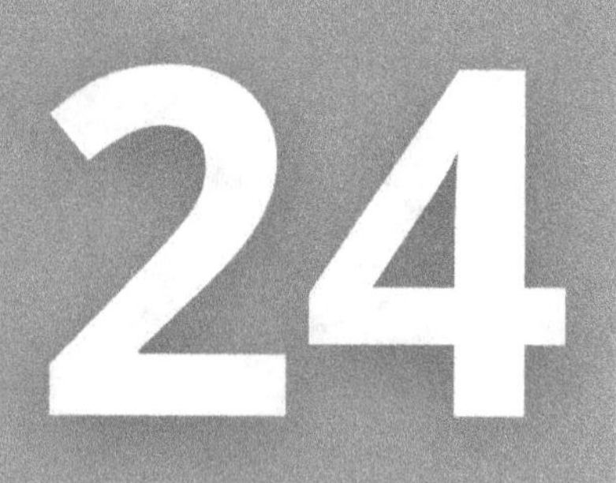

24 Single Leg Series
(Right, Left)

The Single Leg Series exercise stretches your adductor muscles and opens the hips.

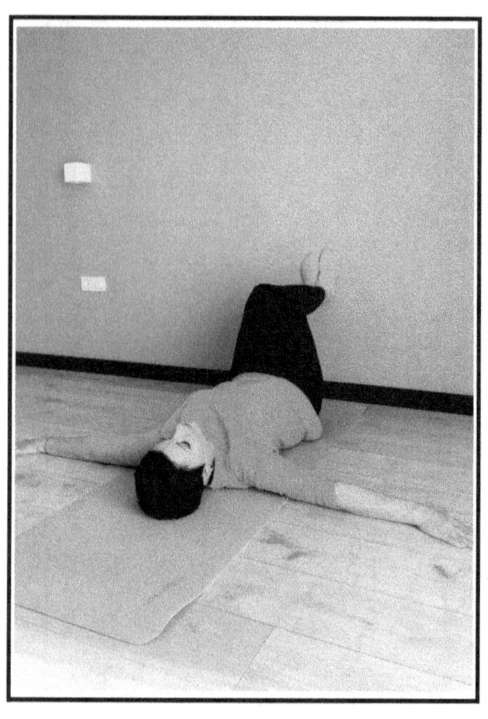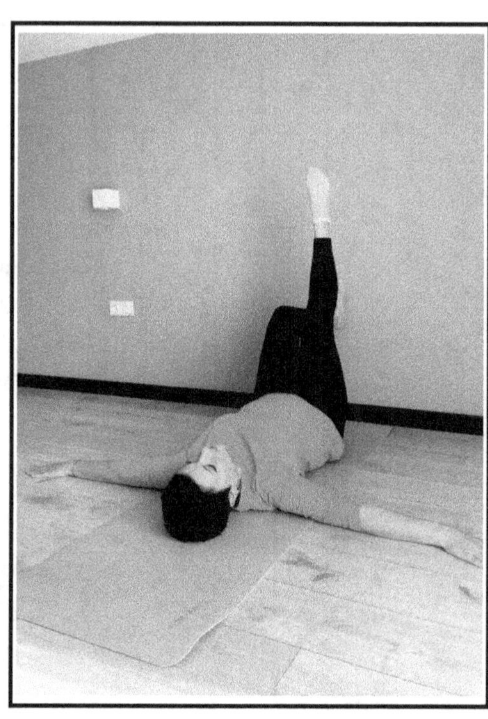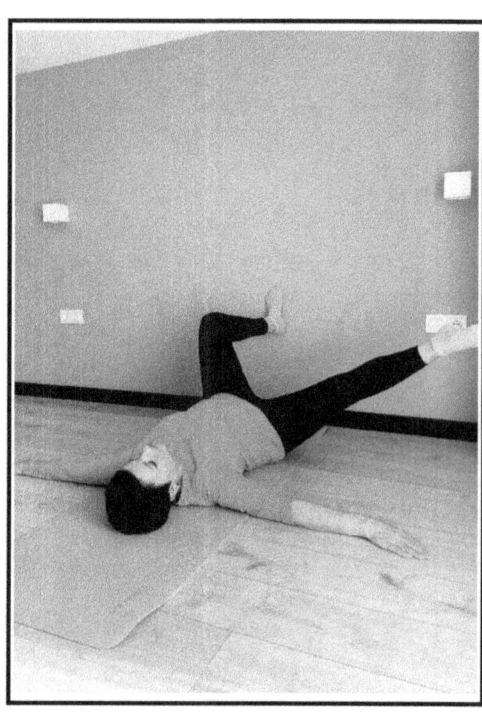

PROCEDURE:

1. Lay down on your back
2. Put your knees at a 90-degree angle on the wall
3. Extend the right leg up, and bring it down to the right side without moving the pelvis
4. Return to the starting position; repeat
5. Perform the same exercise with the other leg

SUGGESTED TIPS:

- Don't bend the leg
- Don't let the leg fall to the side without control
- Don't move the pelvis
- At the beginning of exercise, inhale; as you start to bring the leg down, slowly exhale

Wall Feet Activation

The Wall Feet Activation is an exercise that dynamically stretches the gastrocnemius muscle and tibialis (two large muscle groups in the calves). If you have tight calves, this exercise is a must!

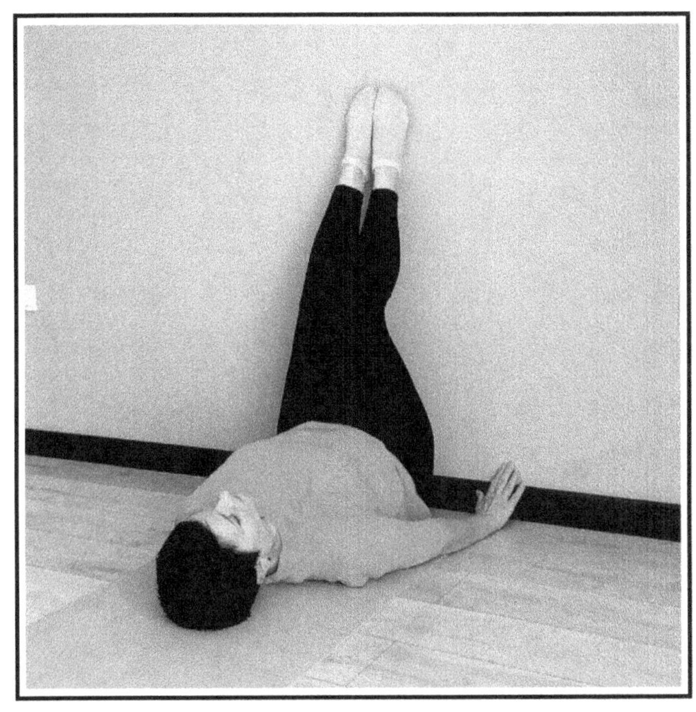

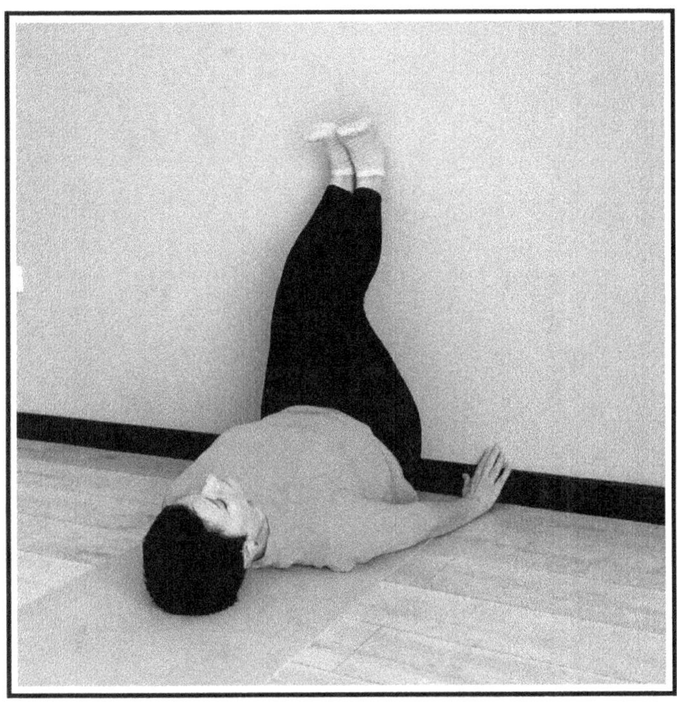

PROCEDURE:

1. Lay down on your back
2. Place the heels on the wall with your toes curved toward you
3. Bend the knees gently
4. Extend the knees while having your entire foot touch the wall
5. Repeat the exercise

SUGGESTED TIPS:

- Don't arch the lower back
- Continue breathing throughout the exercise (maintain a steady breathing pattern)

26 Wall Sit

The Wall Sit exercises strengthen the quadriceps tendon, quadriceps, and glutes.

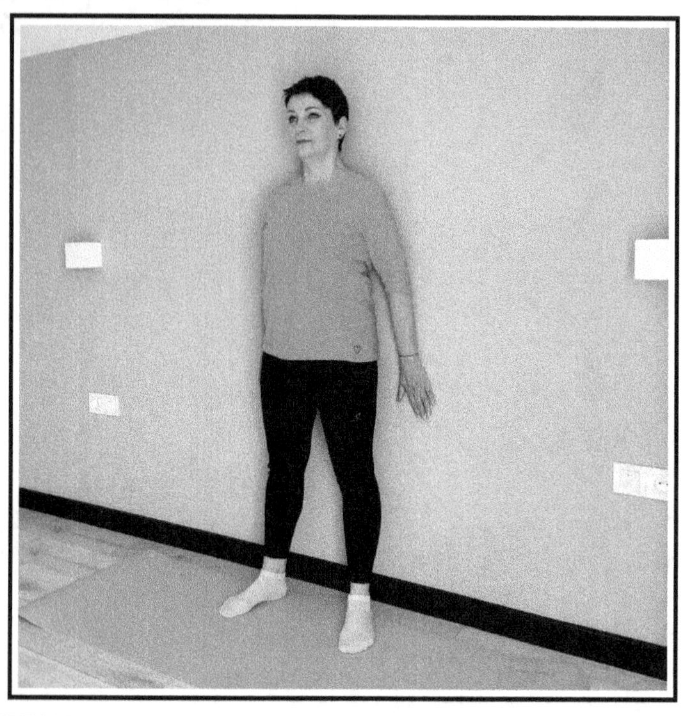 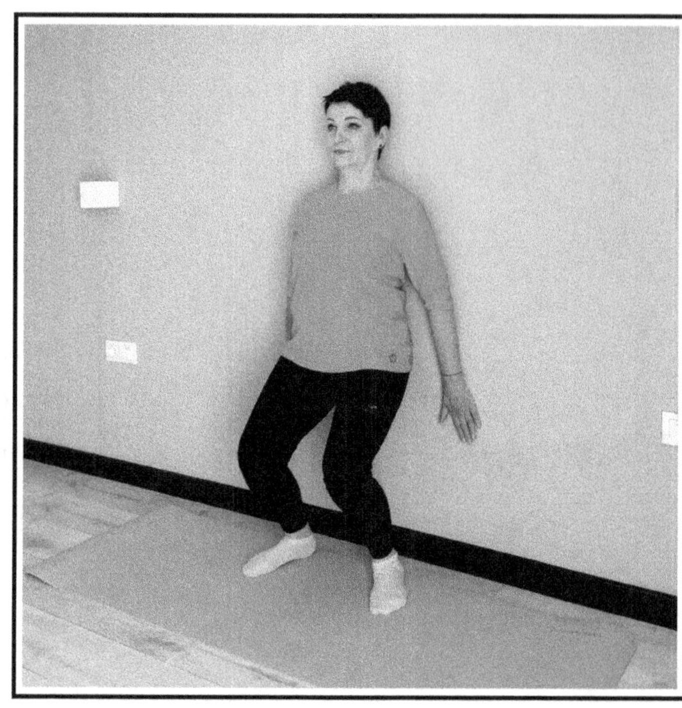

PROCEDURE:

1. Stand up tall with feet about one foot from the wall
2. Place the back, head, and glutes against the wall
3. Slide down the wall until the knees are at a 45-degree angle
4. Hold the static position as long as you can
5. Slide back up the wall

SUGGESTED TIPS:

- Don't go too low
- Make sure to bend your knees
- Keep breathing throughout the exercise
- Keep the posterior chain against the wall
- To make the exercise more challenging, bend the knees to a 90-degree angle

Supported Semi Lunge
(Right, Left)

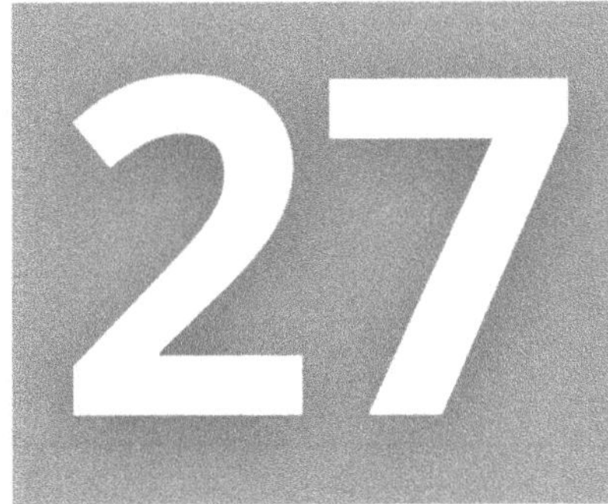

The Supported Semi Lunge exercise strengthens the legs. If you are undergoing strength imbalance in your legs, this is a great exercise for you!

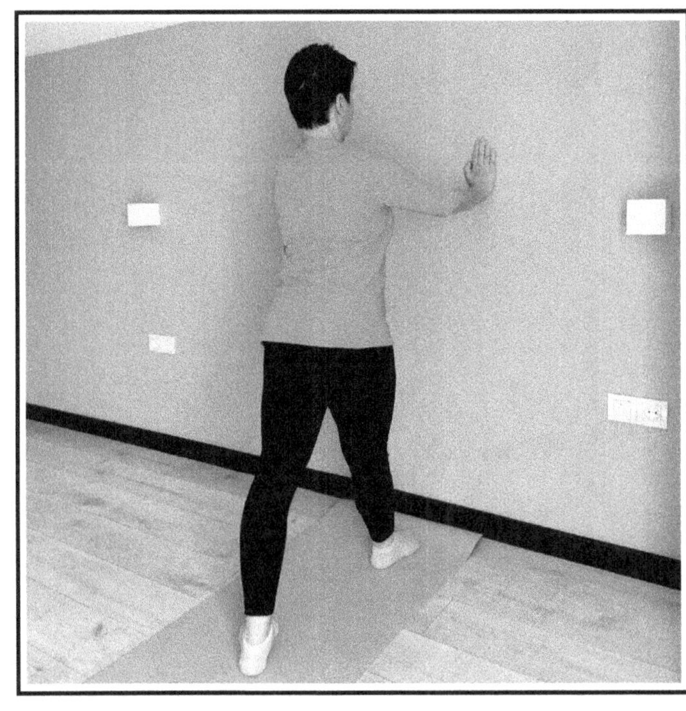
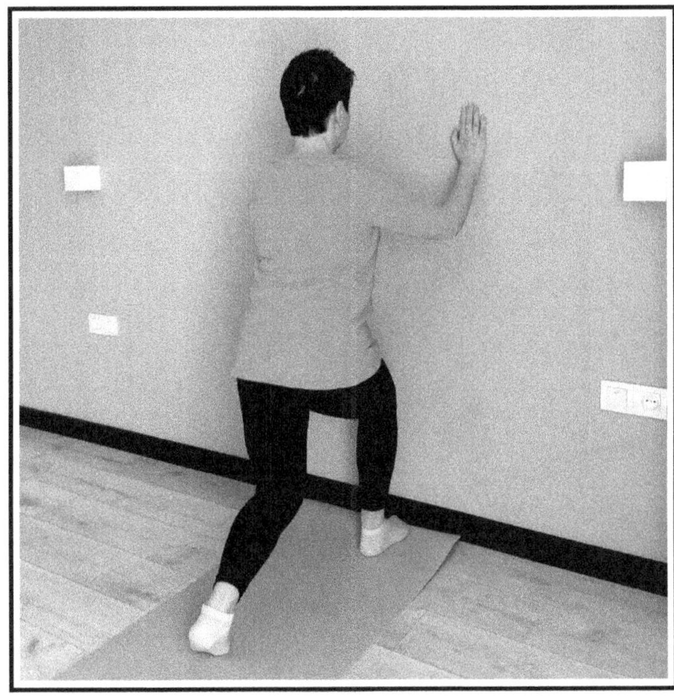

1. Place the hands on the wall
2. Put the left foot forward with toes touching the wall
3. Place the right foot backward
4. Lean a bit forward and bend both legs at 45 degrees
5. Straighten your legs; repeat the movement
6. Perform the same exercise with the other leg

- Don't go too low
- Keep breathing throughout the exercise
- Don't move quickly
- At the beginning of the exercise, inhale; as the exercise continues, exhale

Side-to-Side Lunge

The Side-to-Side Lunge exercise works on the gluteus muscles and quadriceps. The exercise will condition the quadriceps tendons and patellar (kneecap) for more challenging lunge variations.

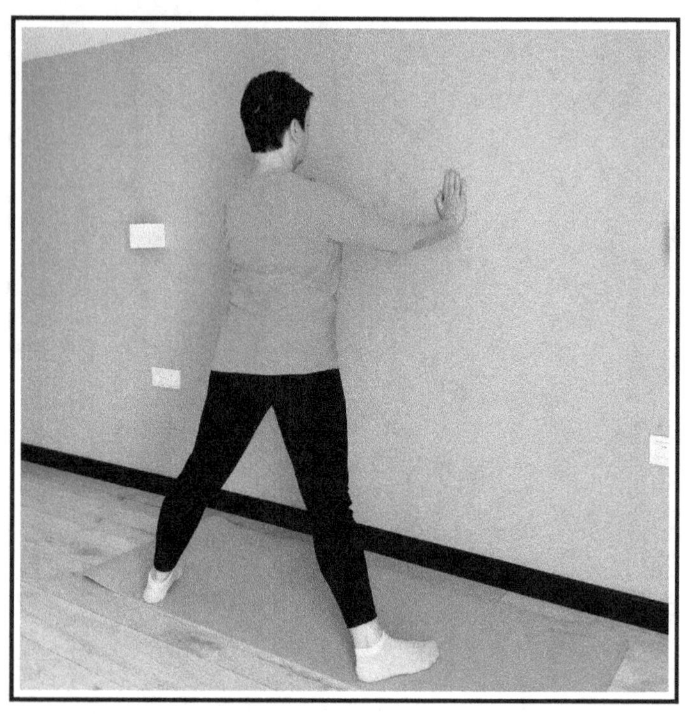
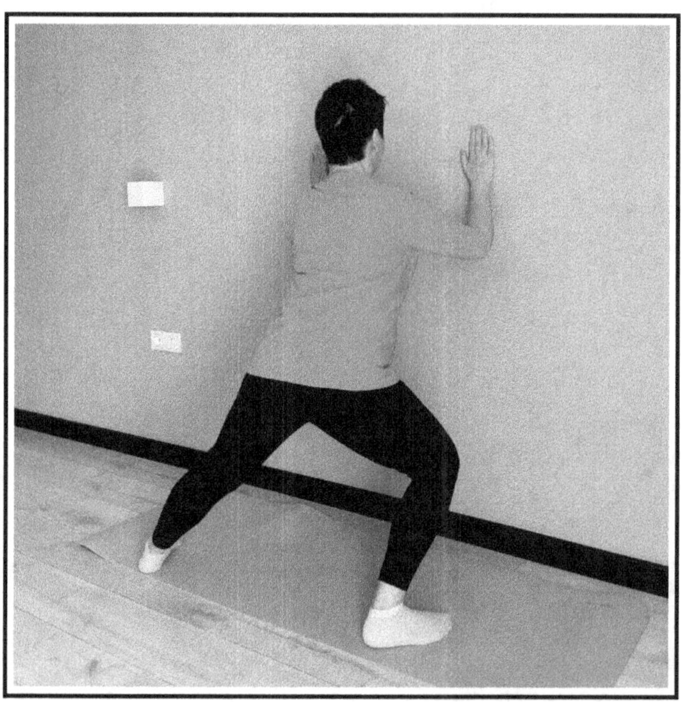

PROCEDURE:

1. Stand with your feet wide
2. Place the hands on the wall for support
3. Point toes outward
4. Bend one knee at a 90-degree angle toward one side; go back up
5. Alternate between sides

SUGGESTED TIPS:

- Don't move too quickly
- Remember to bend the knees at a 90-degree angle

Belly Exercises

29 Crunch Pulses

Crunch Pulses engage the abdominal muscles.

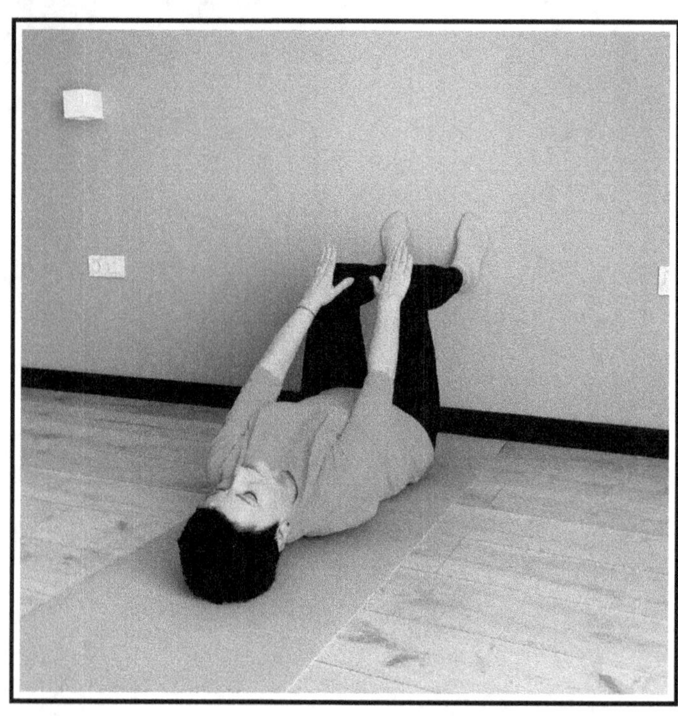

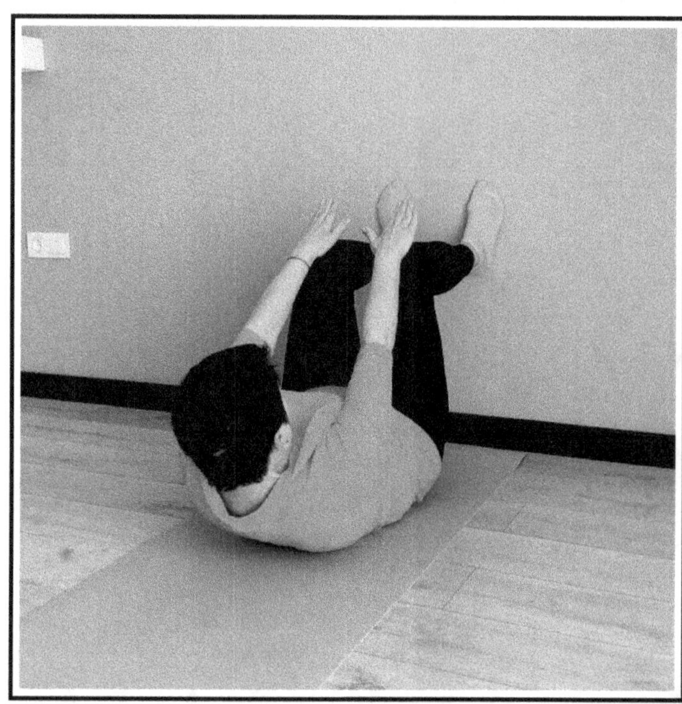

1. Lay down on your back
2. Keep knees bent at 90 degrees on the wall
3. Place the hands on the thighs
4. Tighten the abdominals while raising the shoulders off the floor
5. Move your hands, reaching past your knees
6. Go back up; repeat the exercise

- Make sure to lift the shoulders off the floor
- Move slowly
- Continue breathing throughout the exercise
- At the beginning of the exercise, inhale; as you start crunching, slowly exhale (to fully engage the abdominal muscles)

Reach Through Crunch

The Reach Through Crunch Exercise activates the abdominal muscles.

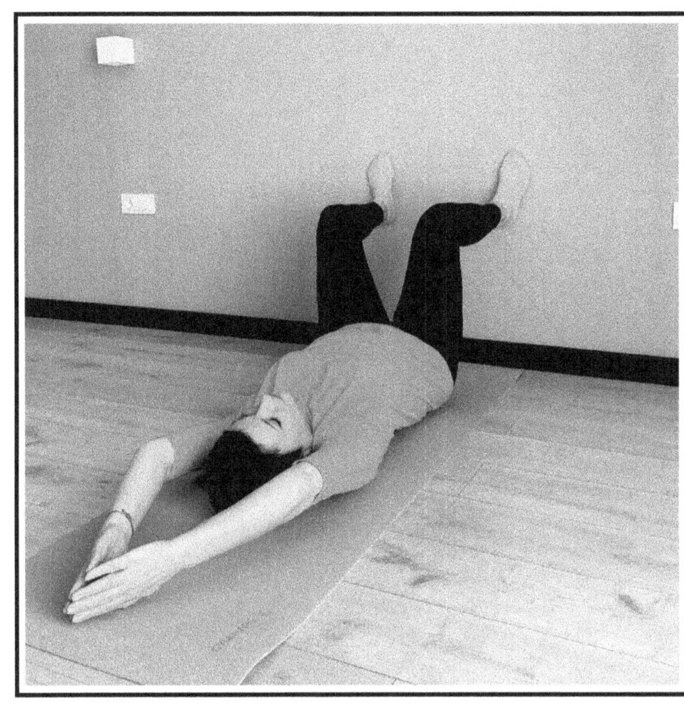

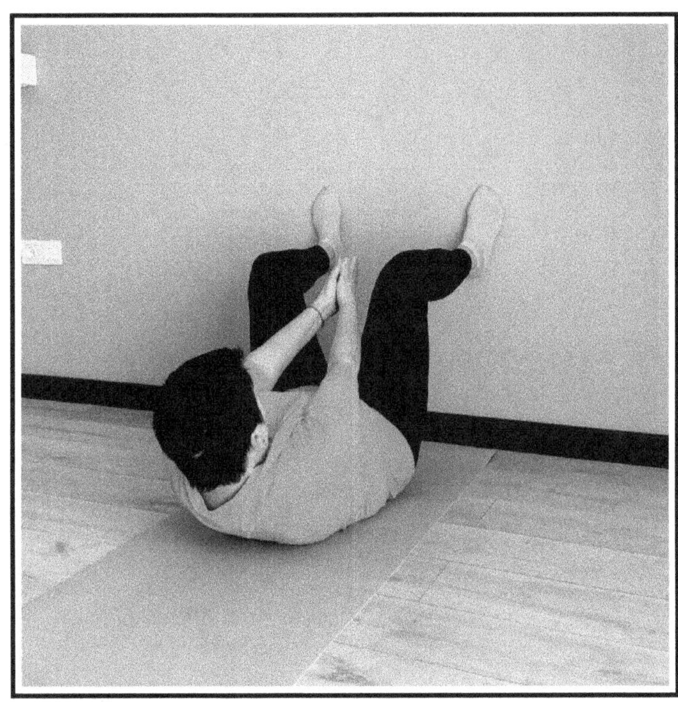

1. Lay down on your back
2. Place the knees on the all at a 90-degree angle
3. Extend arms overhead; put the hands together
4. Contract the abdominals
5. Put your hands between the knees
6. Go back up; repeat the exercise

- Don't arch the lower back
- Remember to lift the shoulders off the floor
- Use momentum
- At the beginning of the exercise, inhale; as you start crunching, exhale (to fully engage the abdominal muscles)

31 Side-to-Side Crunch

The Side-to-Side Crunch Exercise activates the abdominal muscles. It works the rectus abdominis muscle and external oblique abdominal muscles.

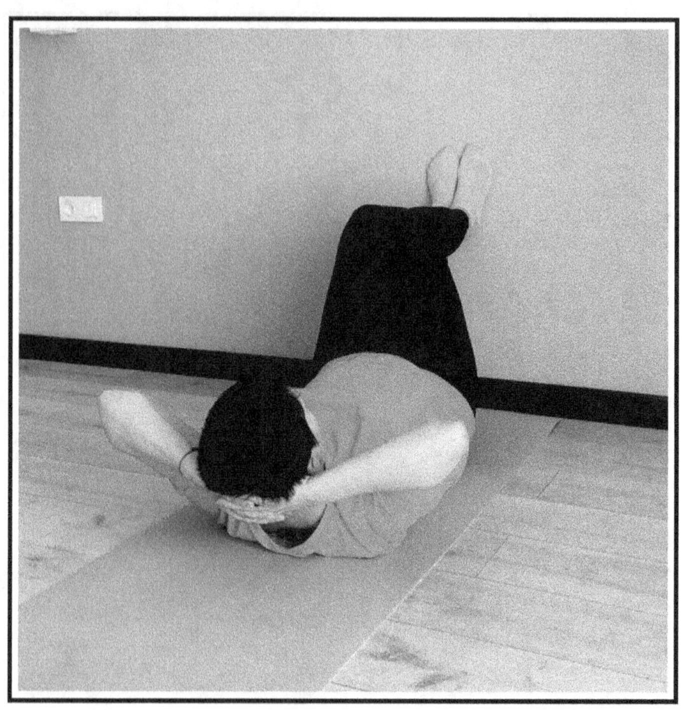

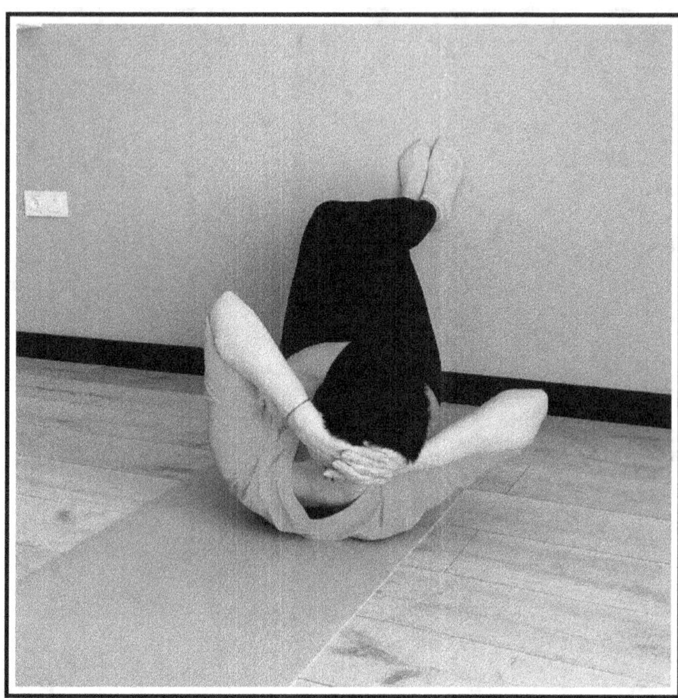

PROCEDURE:

1. Lay down on your back
2. Keep bent knees at a 90-degree angle
3. Place the hands behind the head
4. Raise the shoulders off the floor as you tighten the abdominals
5. Crunch the body over to one side; bring it back
6. Alternate between sides

SUGGESTED TIPS:

- Remember to fully engage the abdominals
- Don't rush through the exercise
- At the beginning of the exercise, inhale; as you start crunching to the side, exhale (to fully engage the abdominal muscles)

Tabletop Oblique Twist

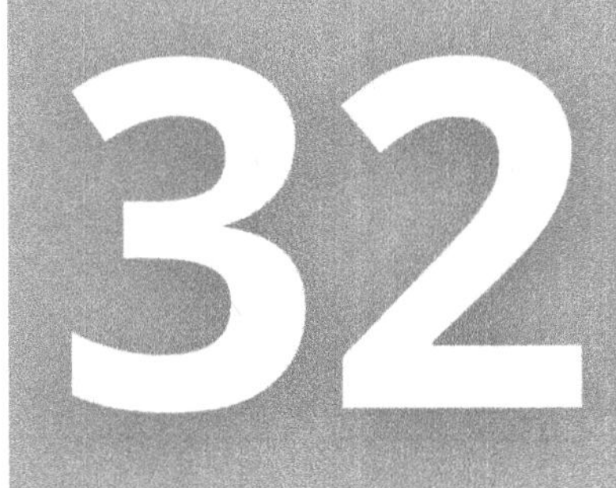

The Tabletop Oblique Twist Exercise activates the abdominal muscles. It works both the front and side parts of the abdominal muscles.

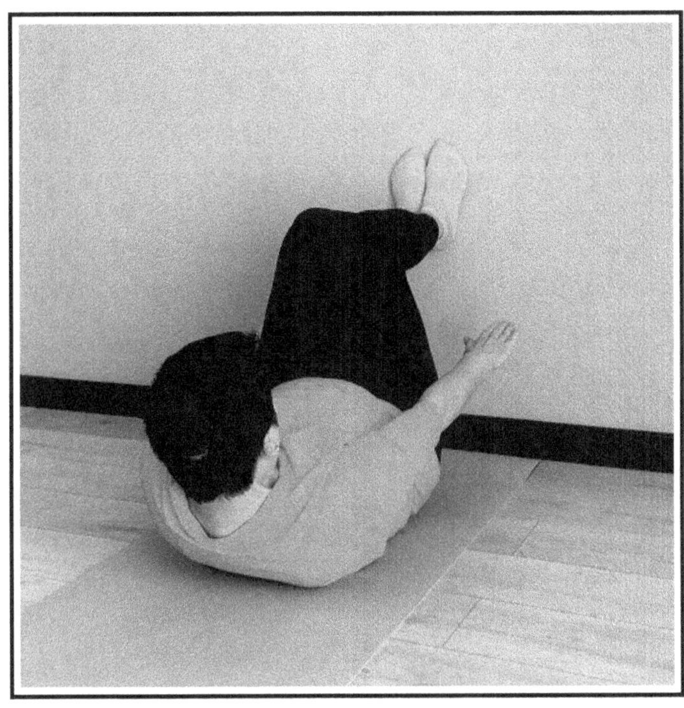 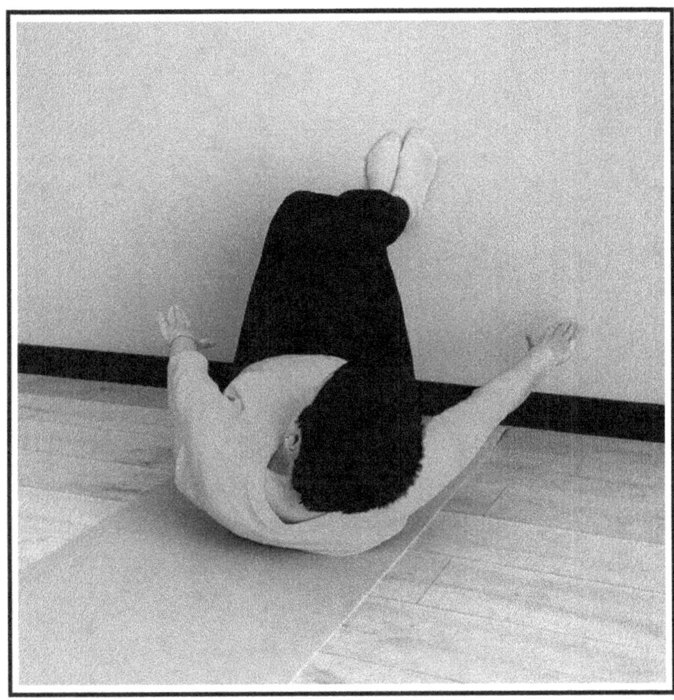

PROCEDURE:

1. SLay down on your back
2. Place the knees on the wall at a 90-degree angle
3. Extend the hands forward and activate the abdominals
4. Crunch the body over to one side; bring it back
5. Alternate between sides

SUGGESTED TIPS:

- Lift the shoulders off the floor
- Don't use momentum (use the abdominals)
- At the beginning of the exercise, inhale; as you start crunching, slowly exhale (to fully engage the abdominal muscles)

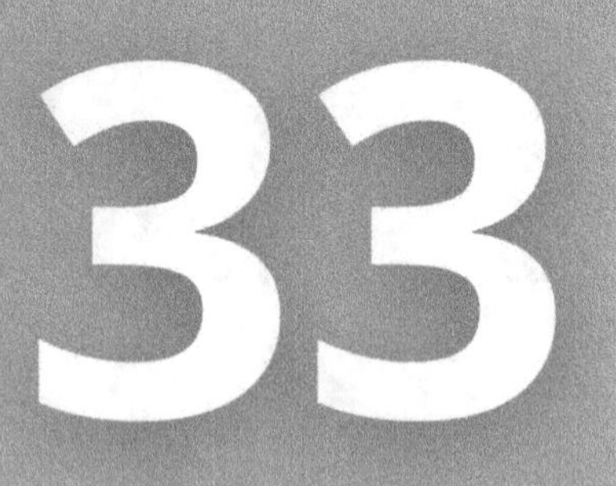

33 Wall Crunch

This exercise activates the stomach muscles and stretches the latissimus dorsi muscle.

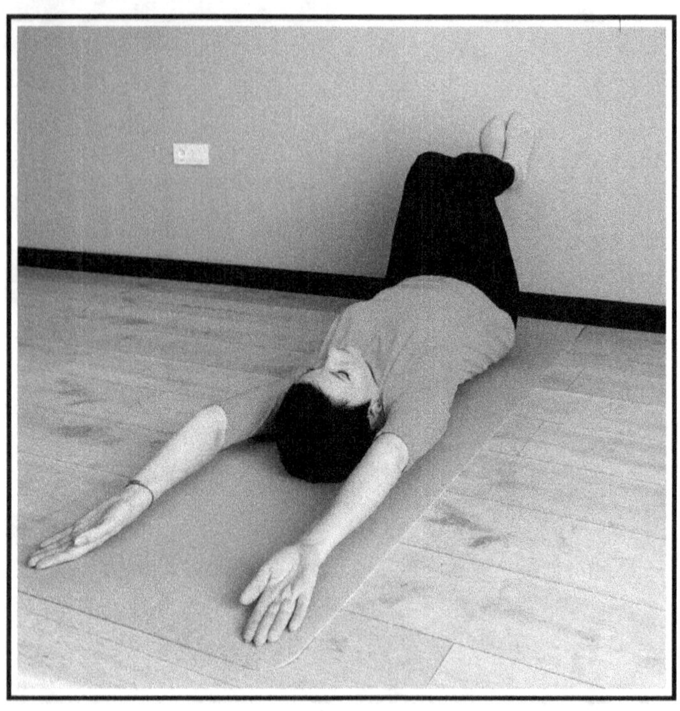

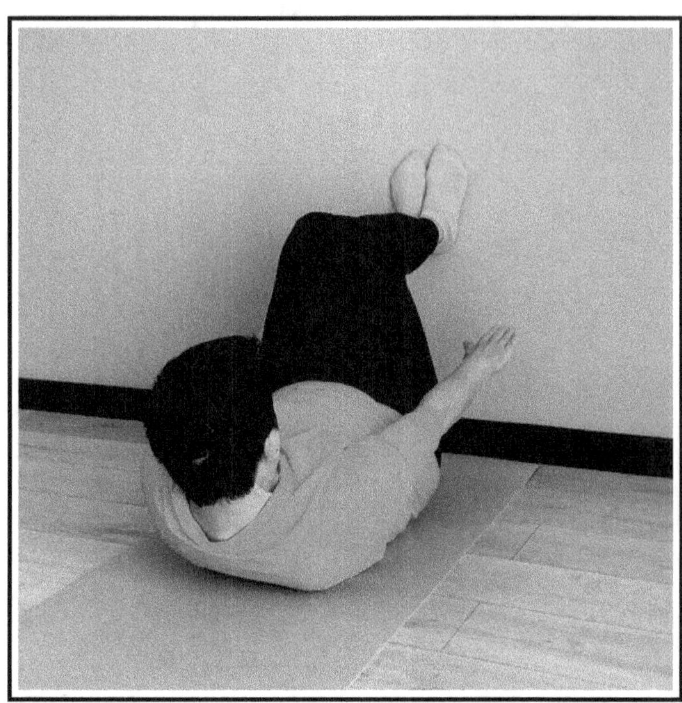

PROCEDURE:

1. Lay down on your back
2. Put your knees on the wall at a 90-degree angle
3. Extend your arms backward next to your head
4. Tighten the abdominals
5. Crunch up; bring the arms forward and let the fingers touch the floor
6. Go back up; repeat the exercise

SUGGESTED TIPS:

- Don't arch the lower back
- Make sure to lift the shoulders off the floor
- Don't use momentum (use the abdominals)
- At the beginning of the exercise, inhale; as you start crunching, slowly exhale (to fully engage the abdominal muscles)

Knee to Chest Crunch

The Knee to Chest Crunch fires up the abdominal muscles and activates the hip flexors.

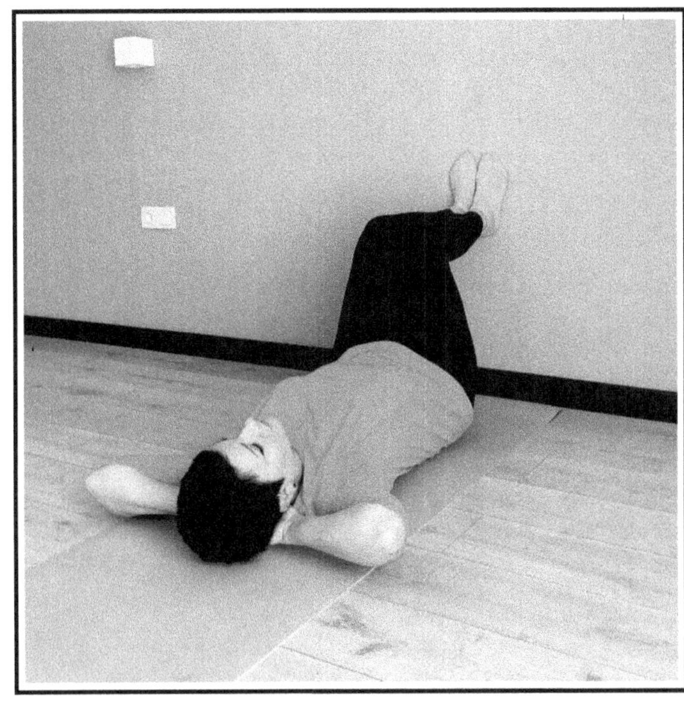 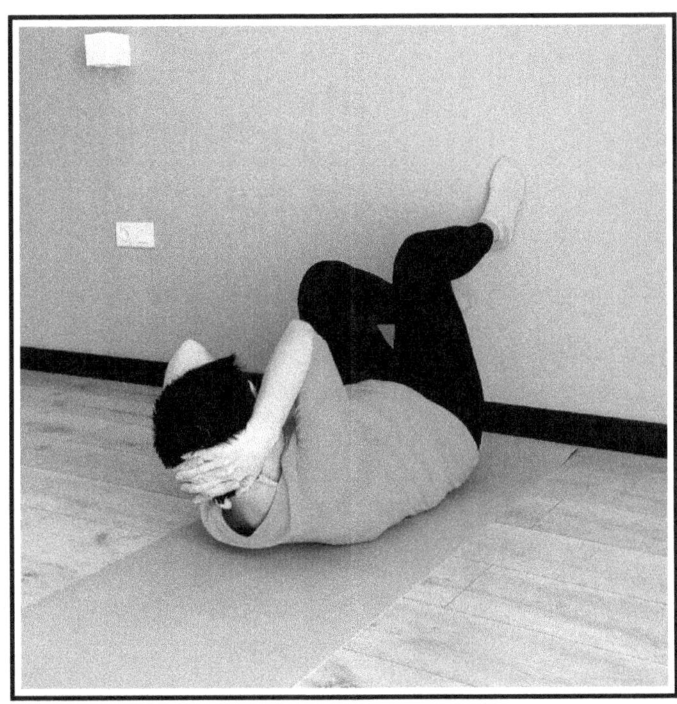

PROCEDURE:

1. Lay down on your back
2. Put your knees on the wall at a 90-degree angle
3. Place the hands behind the head
4. Tighten the abdominals
5. Crunch up while bringing one of the knees to the chest; go back up
6. Alternate between sides

SUGGESTED TIPS:

- Continue to breathe
- Lift the shoulders off the floor
- At the beginning of the exercise, inhale; as you start crunching, slowly exhale (to fully engage the abdominal muscles)

Exercises for Arms, Chest, and Back

Triceps Wall Push-Up

The Triceps Wall Push-Ups condition the tendons for additional and heavier push-up variations. This triceps exercise will strengthen the triceps.

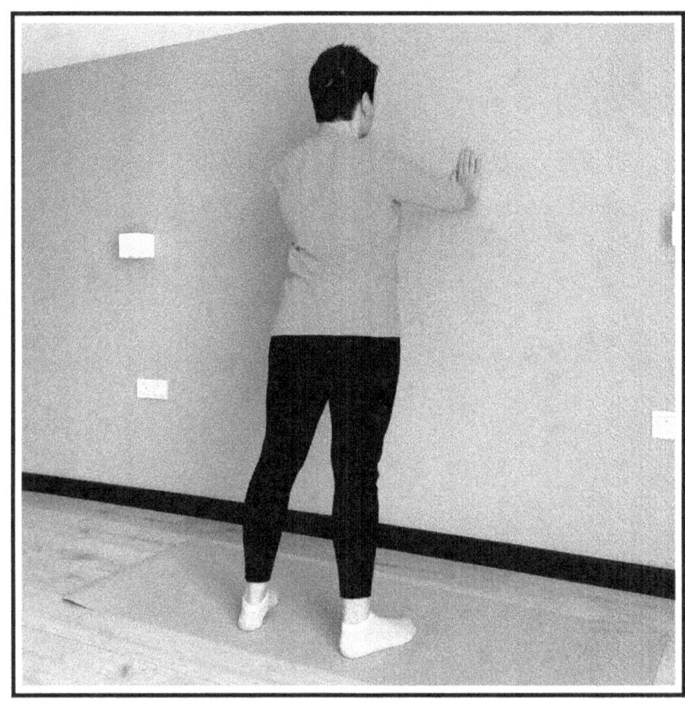 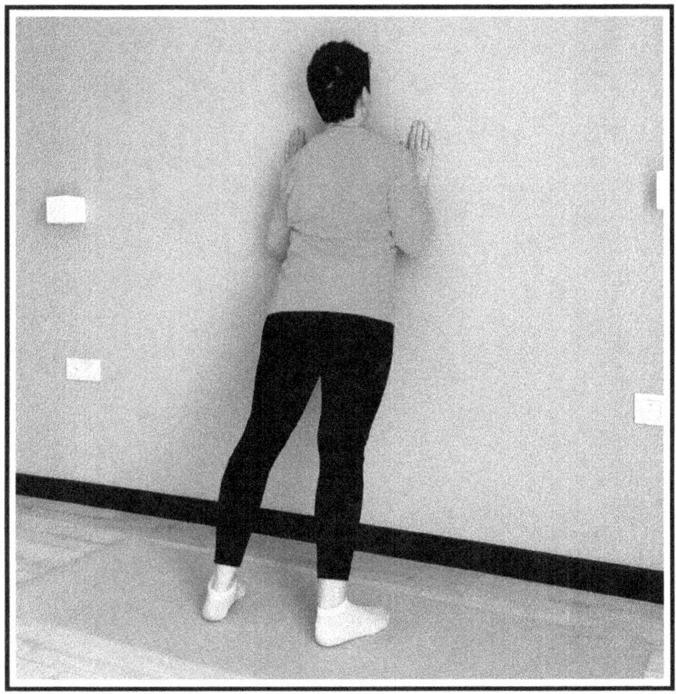

1. Stand up tall with feet spread a little narrower
2. Place hands on the wall at chest level
3. From here, lower yourself until the chest touches the wall
4. Keep your elbows at your side
5. Push up
6. Repeat the exercise

- Make sure to keep the elbows at your side
- Use the full range of motion
- Slower lower the body (as opposed to dropping it)
- Continue to breathe throughout the exercise
- At the beginning of the exercise, inhale; as you push yourself up, slowly exhale

Scapular Retraction & Protraction

The Scapular Retraction & Protraction exercise mobilizes the shoulders, stretches the serratus muscles, and activates the mid-back muscles.

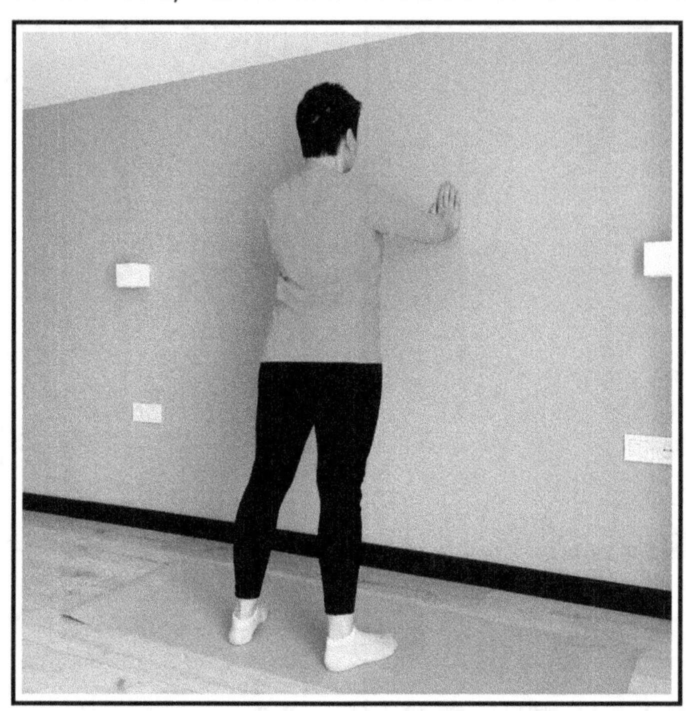

PROCEDURE:

1. Stand up tall with feet spread a little narrower
2. Place hands on the wall at chest level
3. Keep the arms extended
4. Pin the scapulas (shoulder blades) together
5. Push the scapulas apart
6. Repeat the exercise

SUGGESTED TIPS:

- Don't bend the arms
- Move through the exercise slowly
- At the beginning of movement, inhale; as you push the wall, slowly exhale

PAGE 56

Chest Wall Push-Up

The Chest Wall Push-Up exercise will increase the triceps muscles and chest. It will condition the condition the tendons for additional and heavier push-up variations.

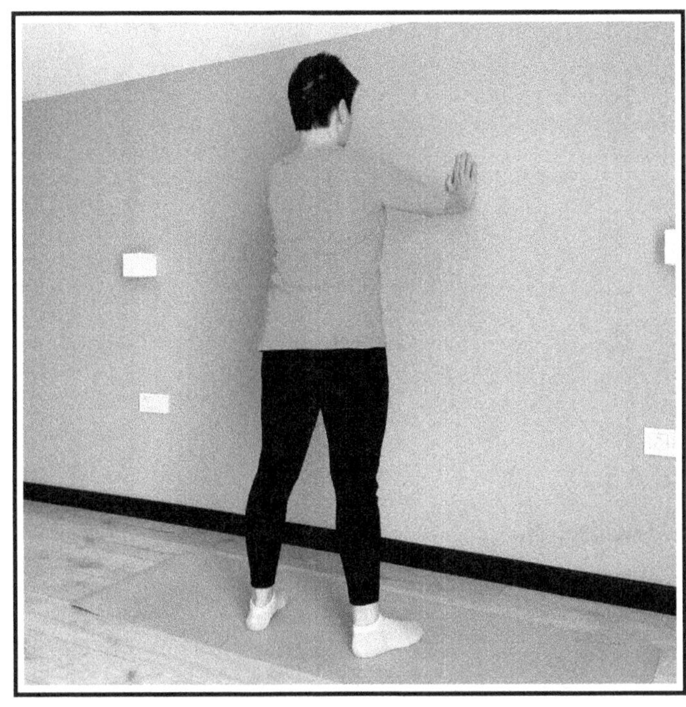

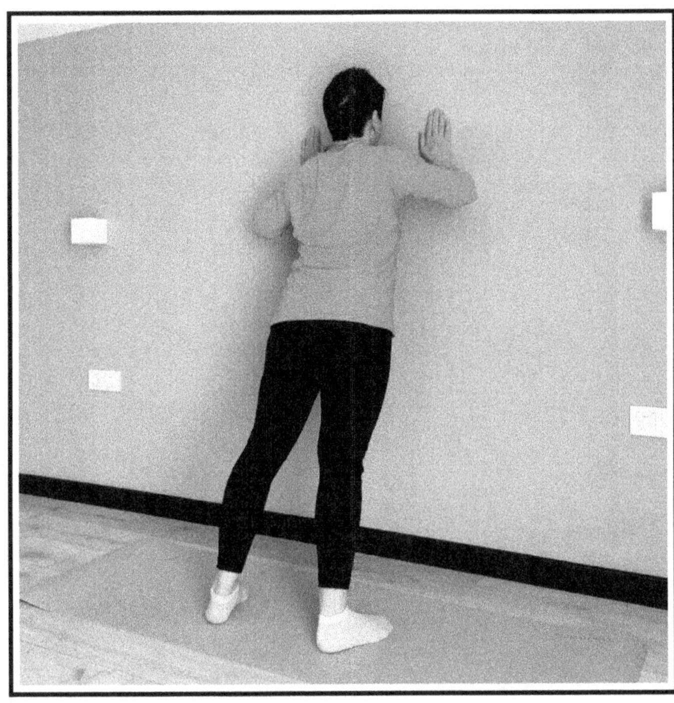

PROCEDURE:

1. Stand up tall with feet spread a little narrower
2. Place the hands on the wall at chest level
3. Lower yourself until the chest touches the wall
4. Keep the elbows at a 45-degree angle
5. Push up
6. Repeat the exercise

SUGGESTED TIPS:

- Stand up tall with feet spread a little narrower
- Place the hands on the wall at chest level
- Lower yourself until the chest touches the wall
- Keep the elbows at a 45-degree angle
- Push up
- Repeat the exercise

38 Chest Openers

Chest Openers do exactly what the name says: they open the chest (i.e., activate the pectoral muscles)

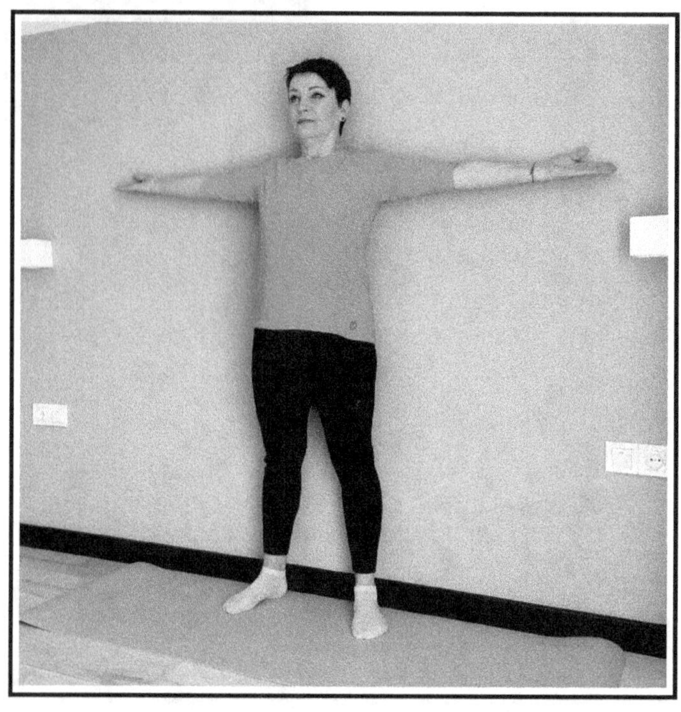

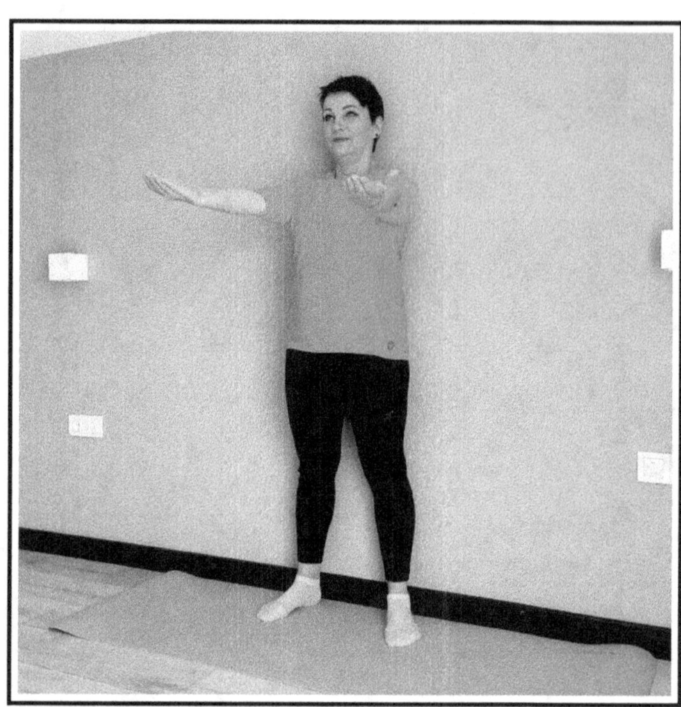

1. Stand up tall with feet spread a little narrower
2. Pin the posterior chain to the wall
3. Extend the arms at a 90-degree angle
4. Rotate the palms toward the ceiling
5. Bring the hands together
6. Move the hands back; repeat the exercise

- Keep the body on the wall
- Continue to breathe throughout the exercise (maintain a steady breathing pattern)
- Don't move too quickly

Robot Arms

Robot Arms is a great exercise to work the rotator cuff muscles and shoulder mobility (internal and external).

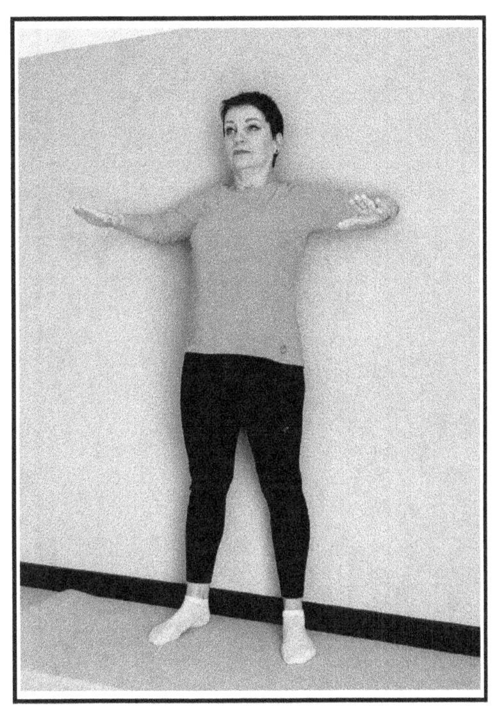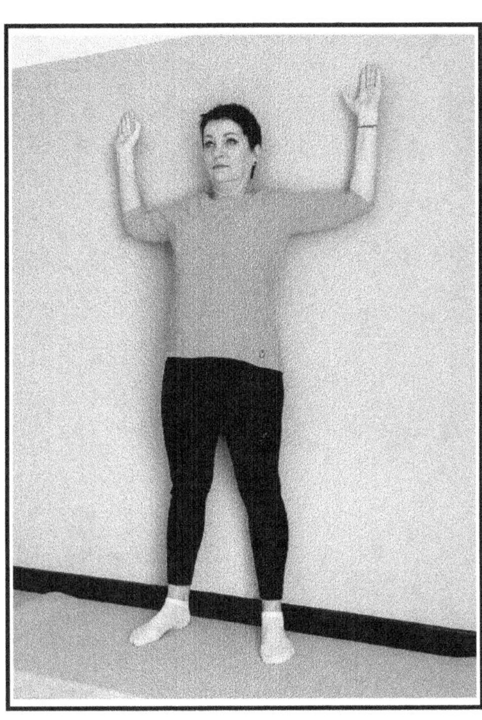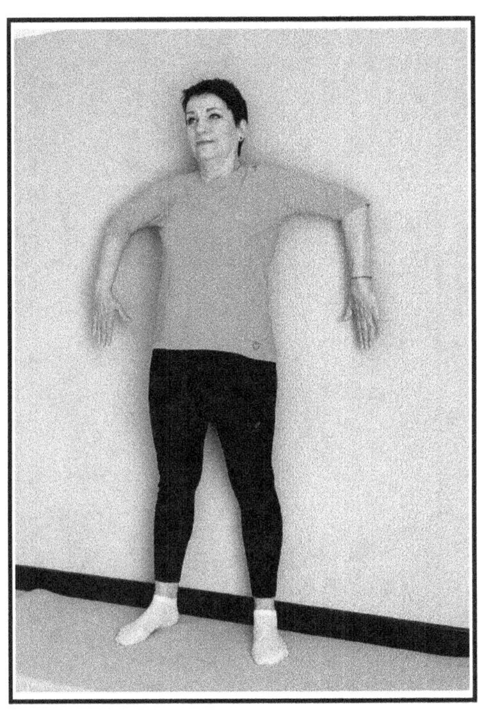

PROCEDURE:

1. Stand up tall against the wall
2. Place the elbows on the wall, at a 90-degree angle
3. Touch the backside of the palms on the wall
4. Rotate the arms down slowly; the front side of your palms will be facing the wall
5. Go back up; repeat the exercise

SUGGESTED TIPS:

- Go slowly
- Keep the elbows on the wall

Wall-Supported Waiter

The Wall-Supported Waiter exercise works the rotator cuff muscles. Note: Chronic shoulder pain can stem from weak rotator cuffs.

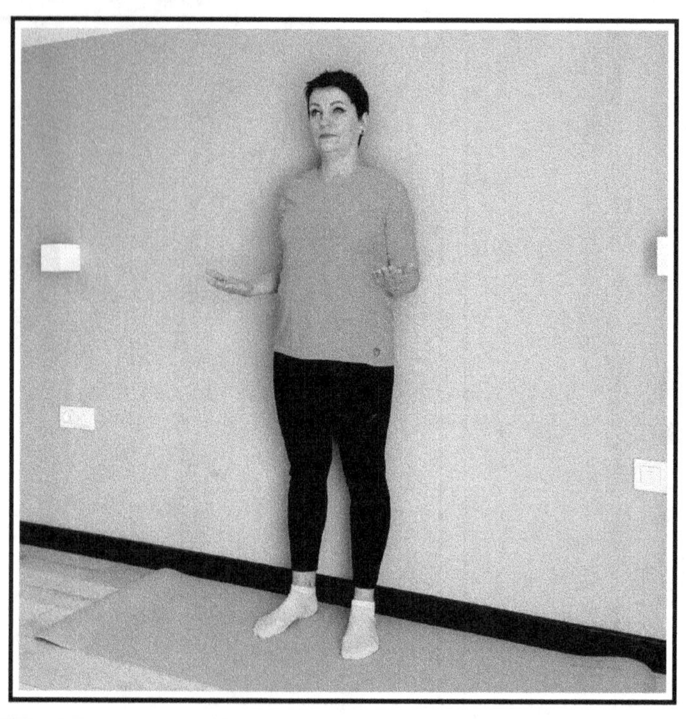

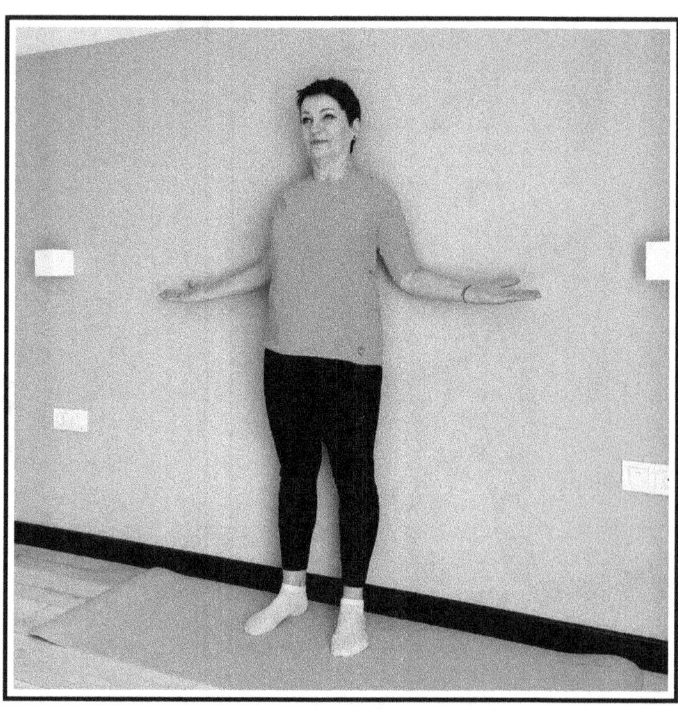

PROCEDURE:

1. Stand up tall against the wall
2. Pin the upper back, elbows, head, and glutes to the wall
3. Bring the hands forward to a 90-degree angle
4. Continue moving the hands to the sides until the thumbs touch the wall
5. Return to the previous position; repeat the exercise

SUGGESTED TIPS:

- Keep the elbows on the wall
- Don't go too quickly
- Keep breathing throughout the exercise

Shoulder Press

The Wall Shoulder Press fires up the mid-back muscles and shoulders, all while improving the posture.

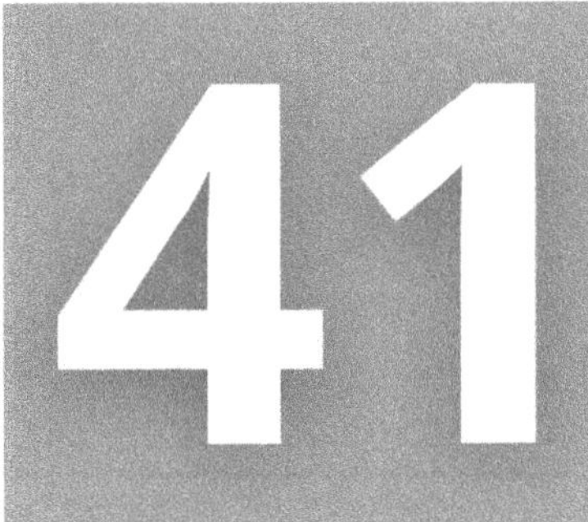

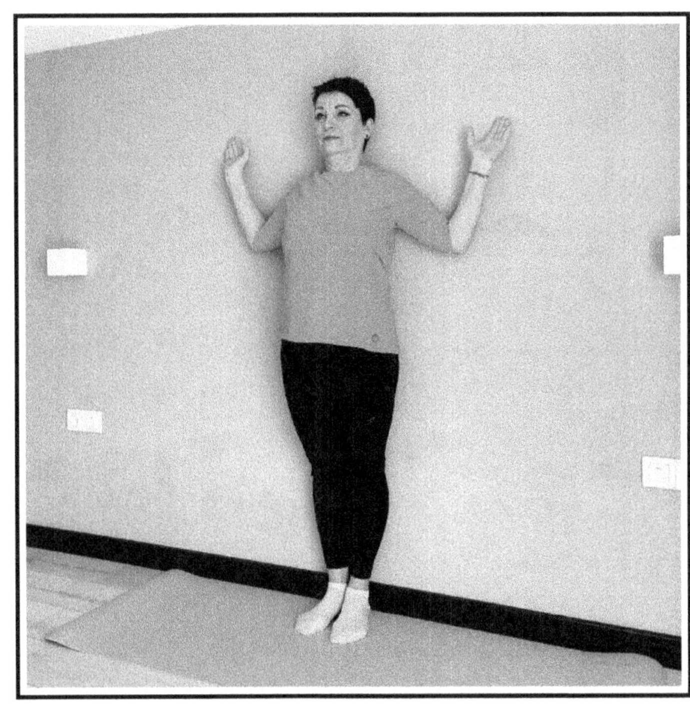 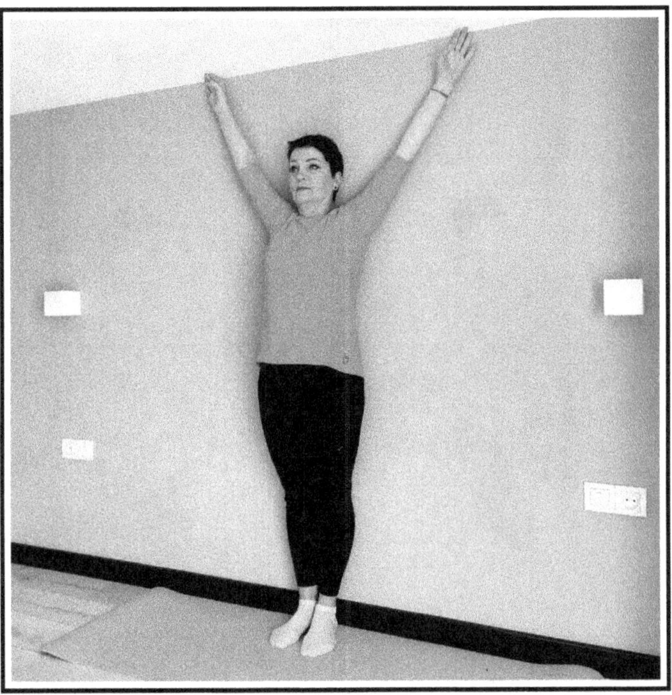

PROCEDURE:

1. Stand up tall against the wall
2. Pin the glutes, head, and upper back to the wall
3. Bend the elbows to a 90-degree angle
4. Slide the arms up
5. Slide the elbows down to the sides
6. Repeat multiple times

SUGGESTED TIPS:

- Keep the elbows on the wall
- Keep breathing throughout the exercise
- Don't go too quickly
- If it's hard to move, take a step away from the wall; bend the knees gently to help flatten the back more

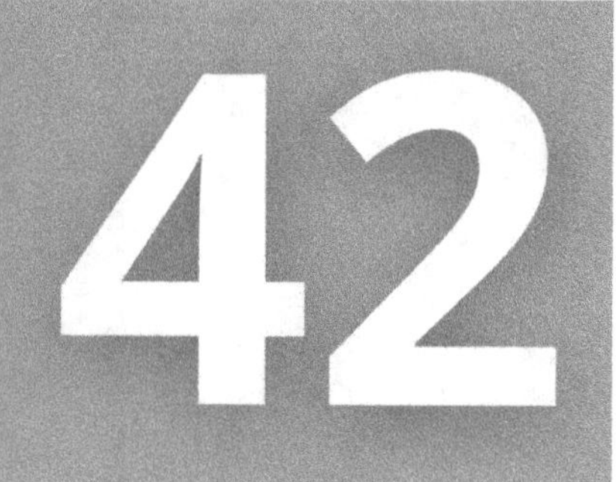

Seated Arm Mobility

The Seated Arm Mobility exercise works on shoulder mobility (internal and external).

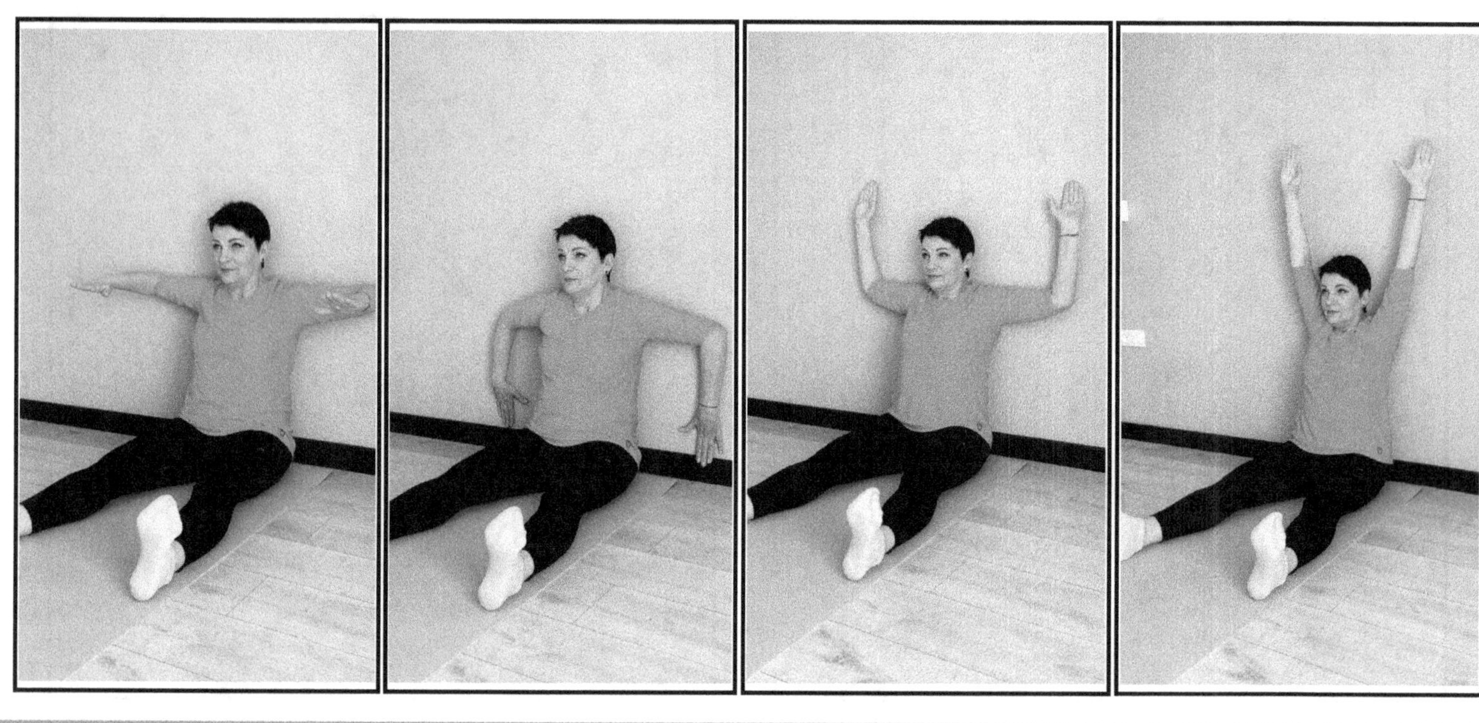

PROCEDURE:

1. Sit up tall against the wall
2. Keep the legs straddled
3. Extend the arms forward
4. Bend the elbows backward to a 90-degree angle
5. Touch the elbows to the wall; rotate the hands down to the wall
6. Rotate the hands up; glide the arms up
7. Extend the arms forward again; repeat the exercise

SUGGESTED TIPS:

- Take your time
- Don't arch the lower back
- Maintain a steady breathing pattern throughout the exercise

Seated Active Forward Fold

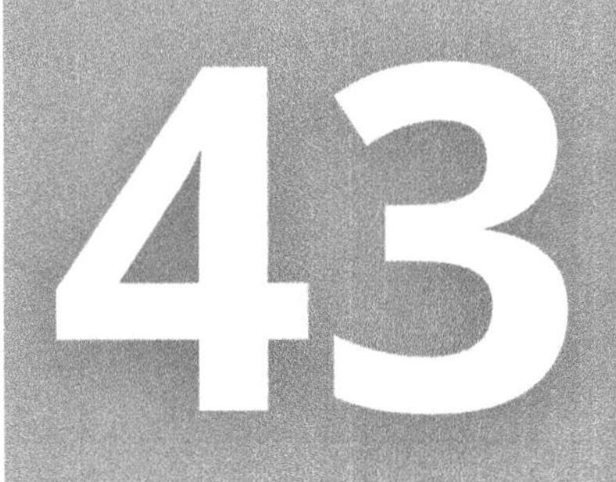

The Seated Active Forward Fold exercise stretches the calf and hamstring muscles; it mobilizes the upper and lower back.

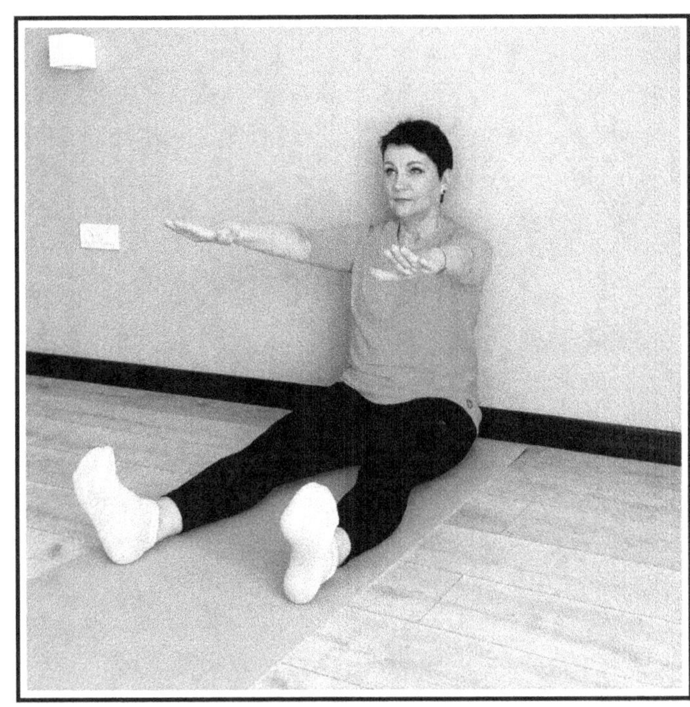

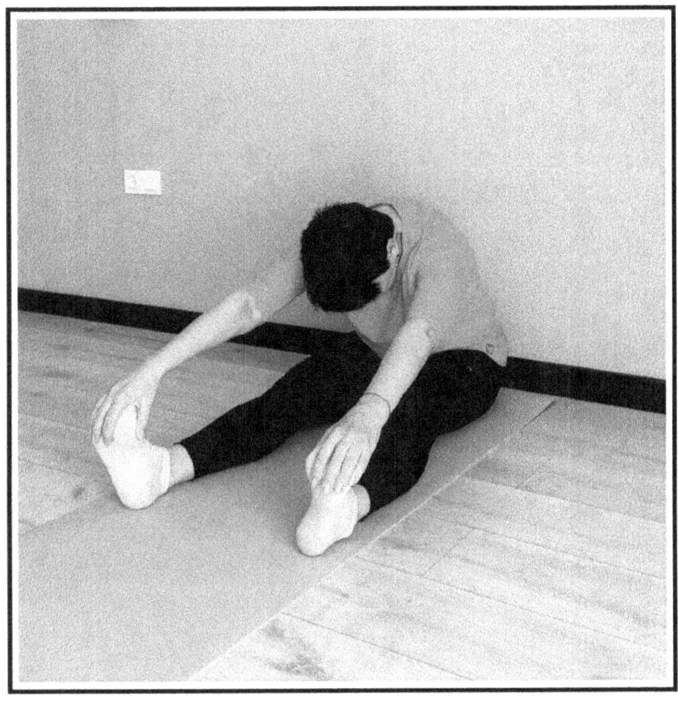

PROCEDURE:

1. Sit tall against the wall
2. Extend the arms up
3. Extend the legs and straddle them
4. Bend the body forward (try to touch the toes with the fingers); hold the stretch for a few seconds
5. Go back up slowly; repeat the exercise

SUGGESTED TIPS:

- Use the full range of motion
- Don't bend the legs or arms
- Maintain a steady breathing pattern throughout the exercise

44 Seated Opposite Toe Reach

The Seated Opposite Toe Reach exercise stretches the spinal erector muscles, hamstrings, and calves.

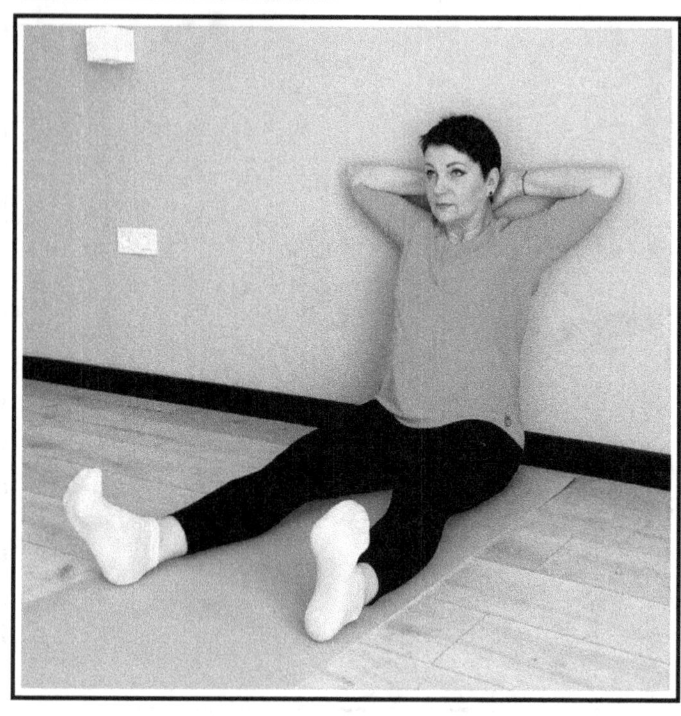

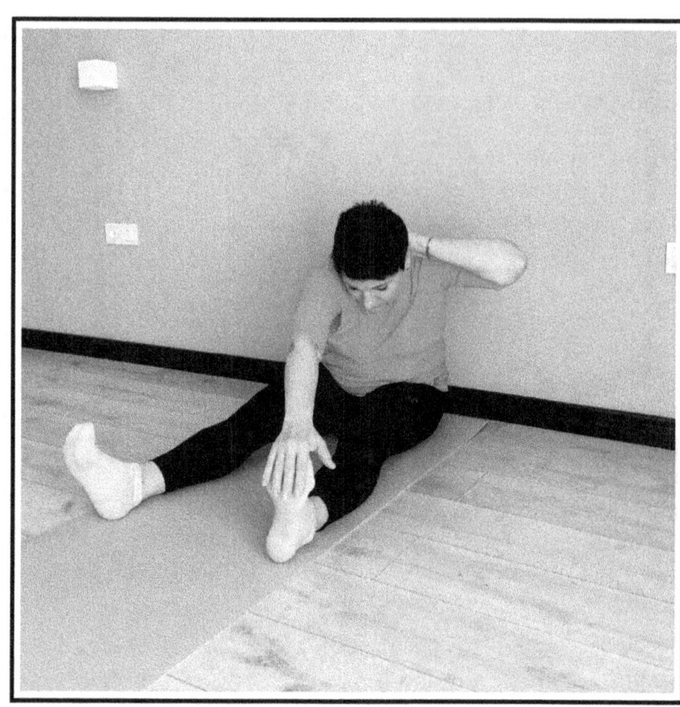

PROCEDURE:

1. Sit up tall against the wall
2. Bend the arms behind the head
3. Keep the legs straddled
4. Reach toward the right toes with the left hand
5. Keep the right arm bent behind the head
6. Go back up
7. Alternate between arms and legs

SUGGESTED TIPS:

- Don't bend the knees
- Maintain a steady breathing pattern throughout the exercise
- At the beginning of the exercise, inhale; as you reach toward the toes, slowly exhale

Supported Roll Down

The Supported Roll Down exercise engages and strengthens the muscles of the lower and upper back. The hamstrings will be stretched a little, as well.

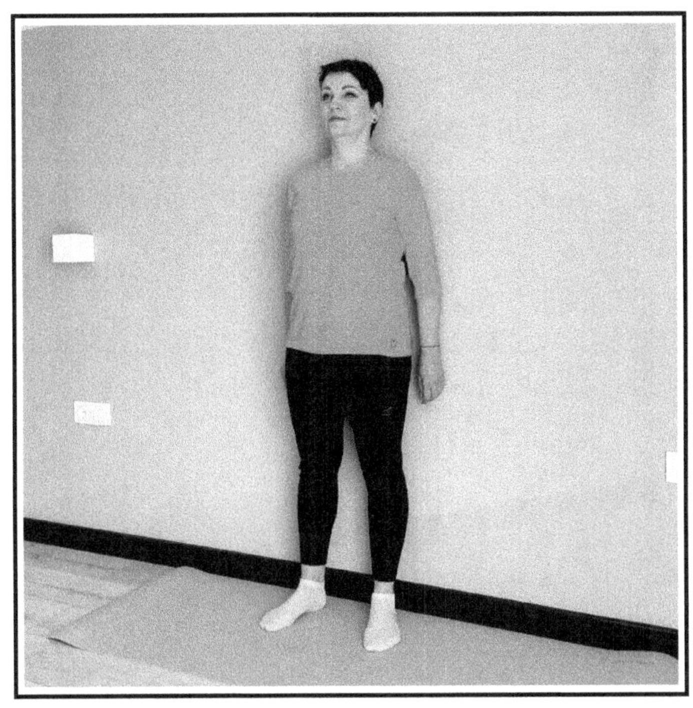 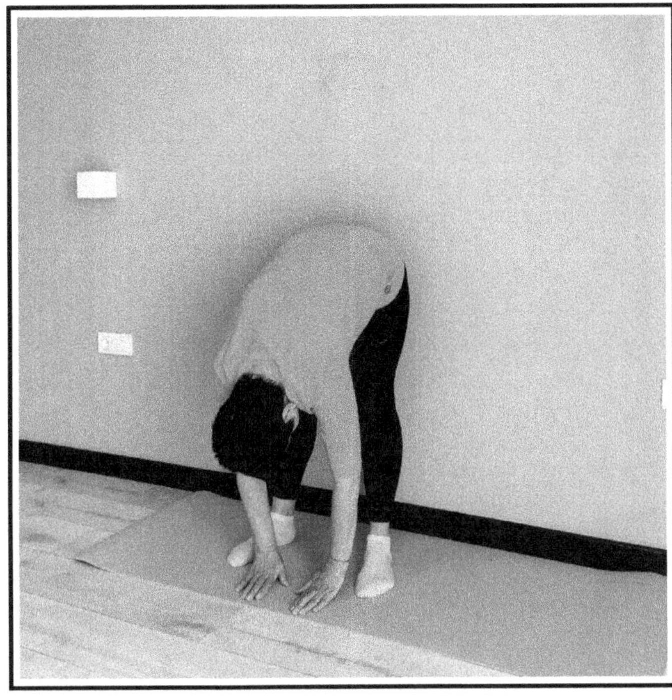

PROCEDURE:

1. Stand up tall with feet spread a little narrower
2. Place the glutes, upper back, and head against the wall
3. Bend the knees gently
4. Begin bending forward (round the head, upper back, and lower back)
5. Relax the arms toward the floor
6. After rounding, stop for a few seconds, go back up, and repeat the exercise

SUGGESTED TIPS:

- Don't bend the knees too much
- Keep breathing throughout the exercise
- Keep the glutes against the wall
- At the beginning of the exercise, inhale; as you start bending forward, exhale

Upper Back Roll

The Upper Back Roll exercise engages and strengthens the muscles of the upper back and stretches the neck. It helps with stiffness in the upper back and neck areas.

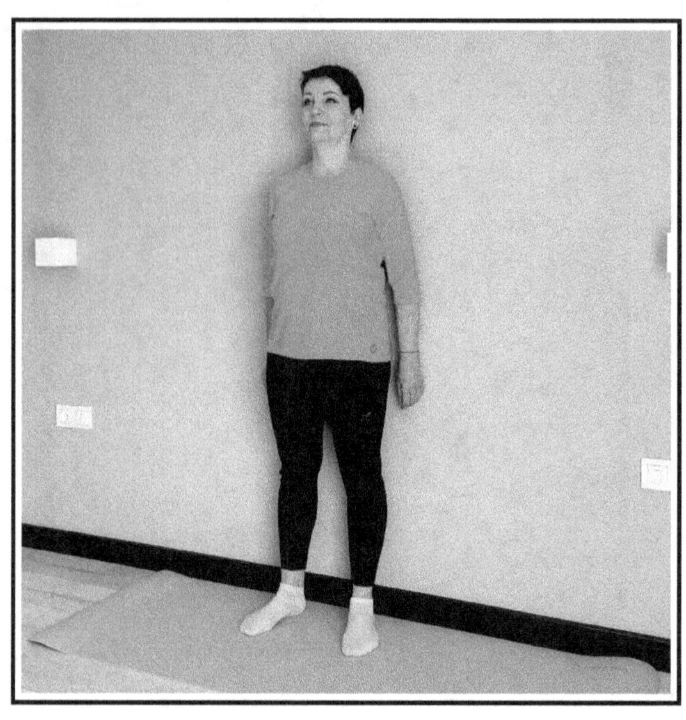
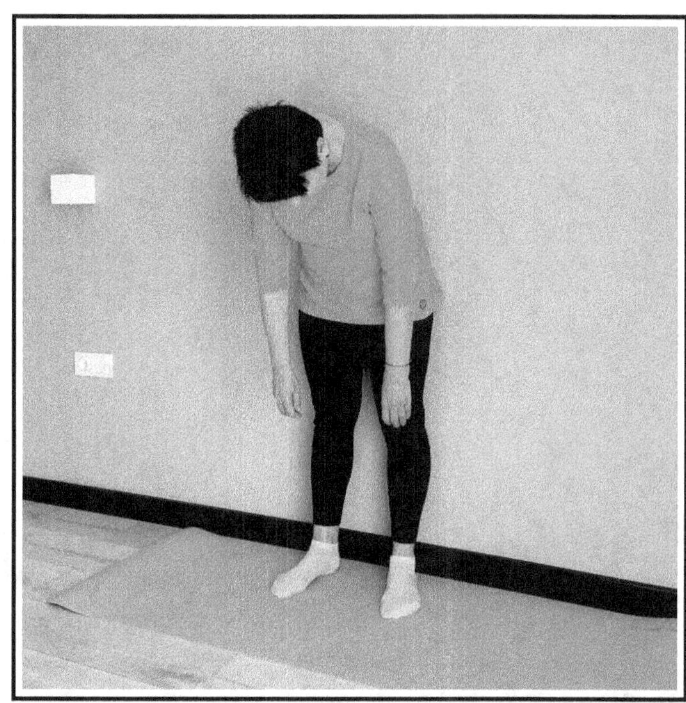

PROCEDURE:

1. Stand up tall with feet spread a little narrower
2. Place upper back, glutes, and head against the wall
3. Keep the knees straight
4. Roll downward by rounding the neck and upper back
5. After rounding, stop for a few seconds, go back up; repeat the exercise

SUGGESTED TIPS:

- Don't round the neck and upper back more than recommended
- Don't bend the knees
- Keep breathing throughout the exercise
- At the beginning of the exercise, inhale; as you start to round the back, slowly exhale

Wall Arms Press Hold
(Palms to the Front, Palms to the Wall)

The Wall Arms Press Hold exercise can make your posture feel more upright and activate the mid-back muscles.

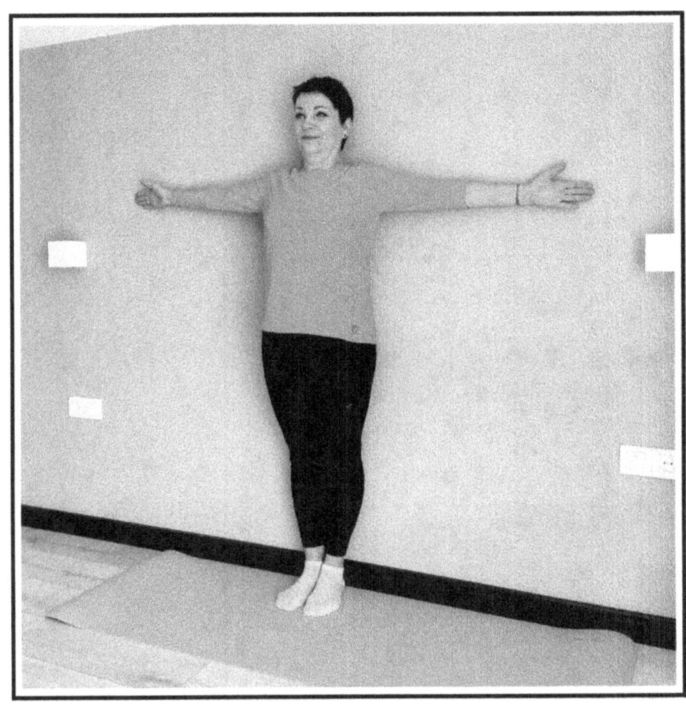

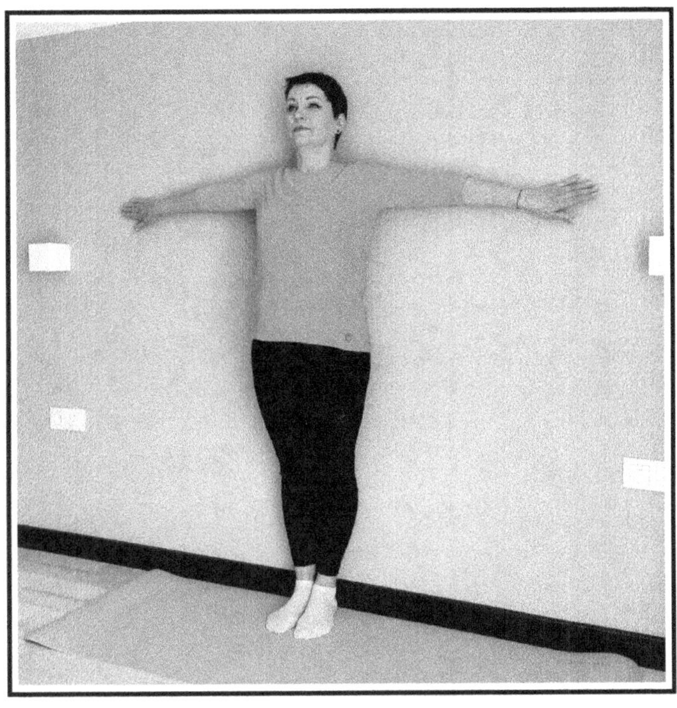

1. Stand up tall against the wall
2. Pin the head, upper back, and glutes against the wall
3. Keep the arms next to the sides
4. Lift the arms sideways to a 90-degree angle
5. With the backside of your palms, press the wall; hold the position
6. Perform the same exercise with the frontside of your palms

- Don't bend the arms
- Keep breathing throughout the exercise
- Keep holding the static position
- At the beginning of the exercise, inhale; as you press the hands against the wall, slowly exhale

Wall-Supported Bird Dog
(Right Arm, Left Arm)

The Bird Dog exercise activates the core and posterior chain. It challenges your stability, too!

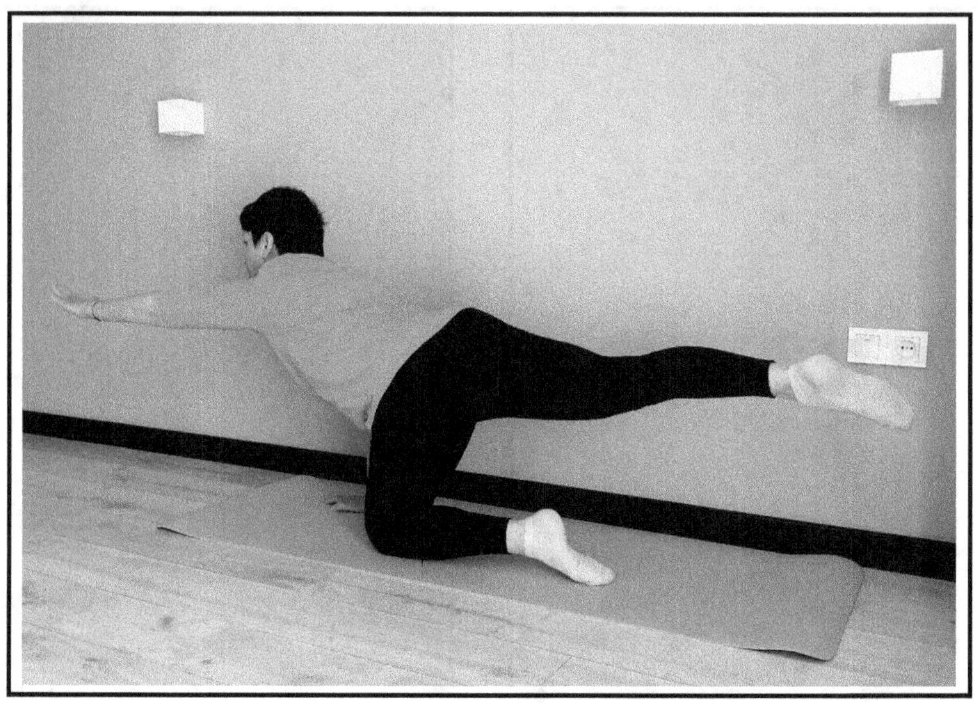

PROCEDURE:

1. Get down on all fours, sideways to the wall
2. Tighten the abdominals
3. Keep the knees under the hips
4. Keep the hands under the shoulders
5. Extend your left arm and your right leg at the same time
6. Hold the static position
7. Repeat the exercise with the other arm and leg

SUGGESTED TIPS:

- Keep the lower back straight
- Don't move too quickly
- Tighten the abdominals before beginning the exercise

Stretching

49

Cross Arm Stretch
(Right on Top, Left on Top)

The Cross Arm Stretch is a great exercise to stretch the triceps, rear, and side deltoid muscles.

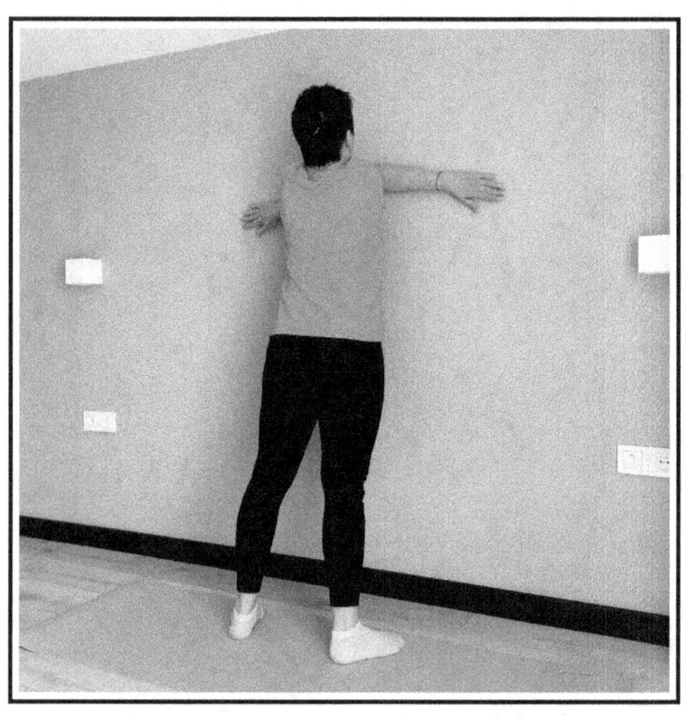

PROCEDURE:

1. Stand tall hip-width apart
2. Place the hands and elbows on the wall; cross them (the right arm over the top)
3. Slide your hands to the side until you start feeling the stretch
4. Hold the stretch
5. Repeat with left arm over the top

SUGGESTED TIPS:

- Keep breathing throughout the exercise (maintain a steady breathing pattern)
- Don't arch the lower back

Alternating Arm Straightening

The Alternating Arm Straightening exercise stretches the neck muscles and the latissimus dorsi muscle (the biggest muscle in the back).

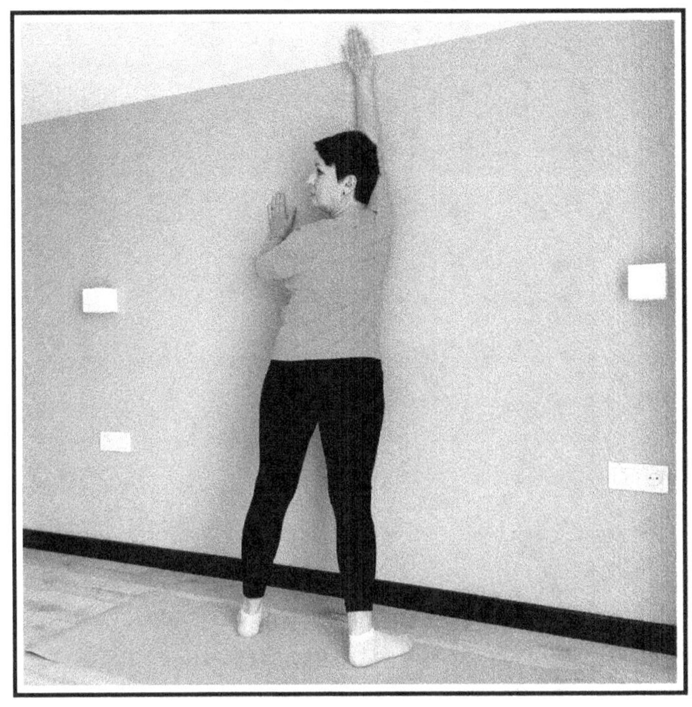 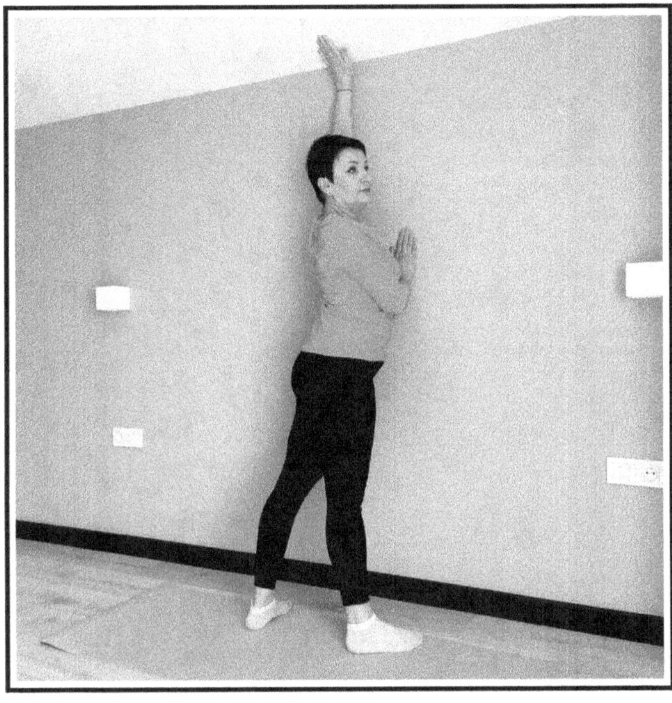

PROCEDURE:

1. Stand tall hip-width apart
2. Place hands on the wall
3. Glide one palm upward until you reach a full arm extension
4. Look away when sliding the hand
5. Hold the stretch
6. Repeat with the other palm upward

SUGGESTED TIPS:

- Don't bend the arm
- Don't arch the lower back
- At the beginning of the movement, inhale; as you glide the palm up, exhale

Forearm Stretch

The Forearm Stretch exercise is a sure way to relax your forearms. The exercise also helps with stiffness in the forearms.

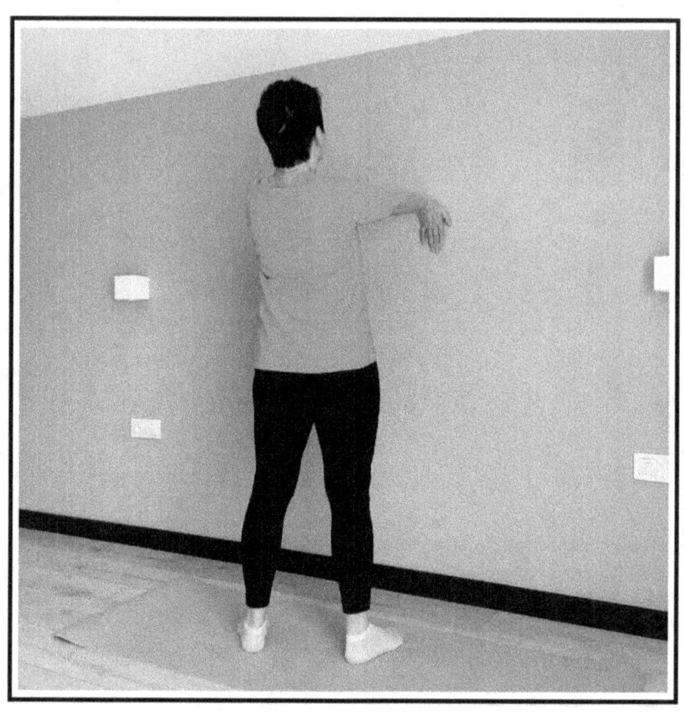

PROCEDURE:

1. Stand up tall
2. Place the feet together
3. Place the hands on the wall (at shoulder level)
4. Turn the fingers downward
5. Keep the arms extended
6. Hold the static stretch

SUGGESTED TIPS:

- Don't bend the arms
- Continue breathing throughout the exercise (maintain a steady breathing pattern)

Alternating Chest Stretch

The Alternating Chest Stretch exercise does just that! It stretches the biceps and the pectoral and deltoid muscles.

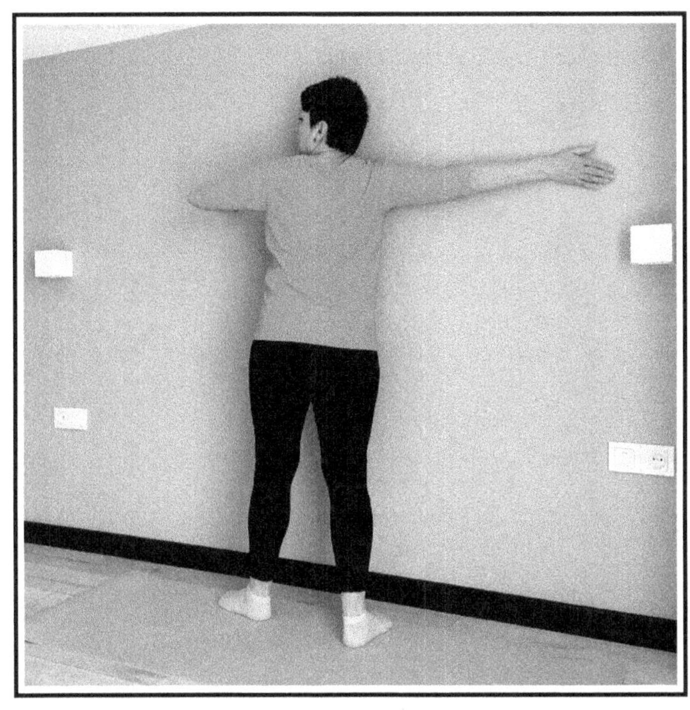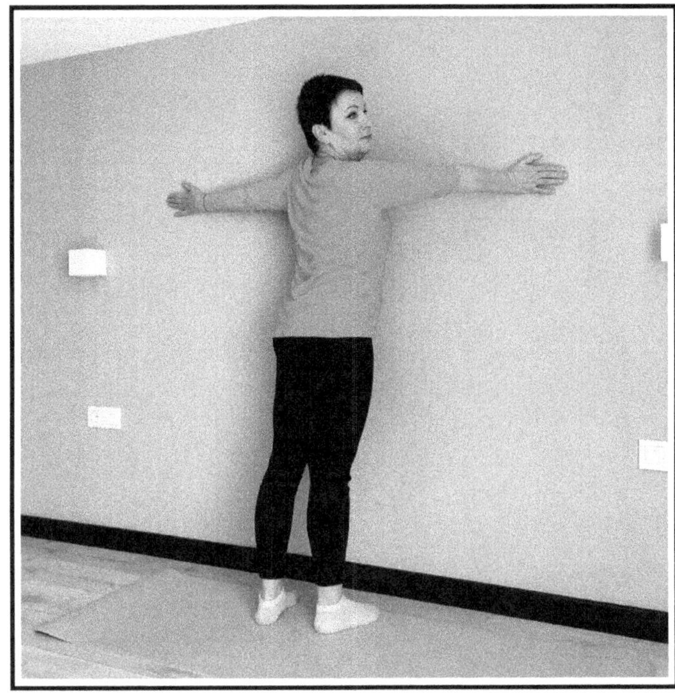

PROCEDURE:

1. Stand tall hip-width apart
2. Open the arms wide and place the hands sideways on the wall
3. Rotate the chest to one arm
4. Bend the arm (you are leaning on), and keep the other arm extended
5. Hold the stretch; repeat with the other arm

SUGGESTED TIPS:

- Do the exercise on both sides
- Don't bend both arms
- Make sure to rotate the chest toward one arm
- At the beginning of the exercise, inhale; as you lean toward the arm, exhale

53 Alternating Arm Reach

The Alternating Arm Reach exercise stretches the latissimus dorsi muscle and the external abdominal muscles (i.e., obliques). It works wonders, especially if you are experiencing stiffness on one side of the body.

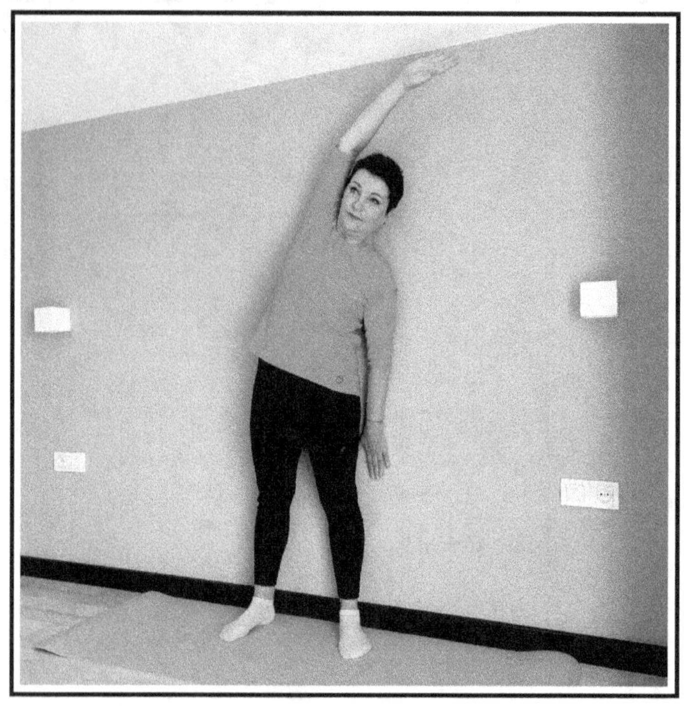

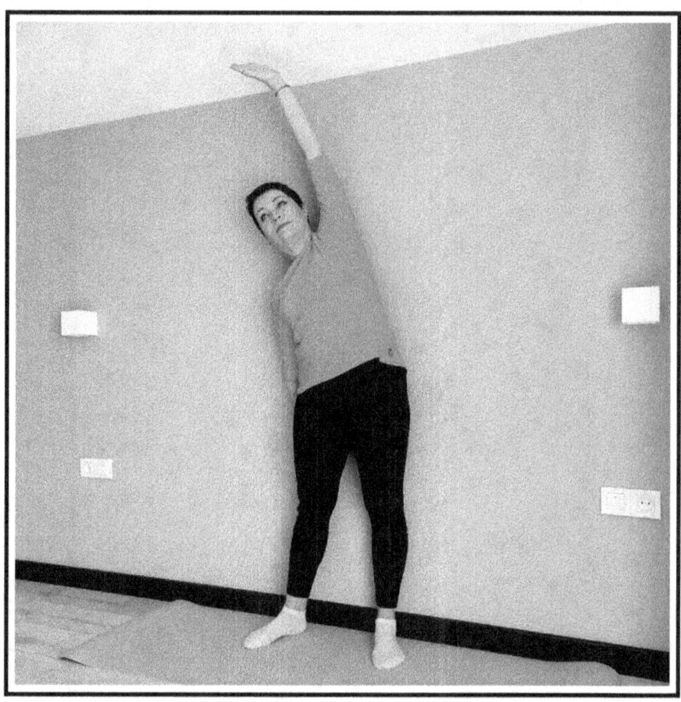

PROCEDURE:

1. Stand up tall against the wall
2. Pin the head, glutes, upper back, and arms against the wall
3. Lift one arm up; reach across the head
4. Keep the arms straight
5. Go back up
6. Alternate between sides

SUGGESTED TIPS:

- Don't bend the arms
- Don't move too quickly
- At the beginning of the exercise, inhale; as you lift the arm across the body, exhale

Split Stance Side Stretch
(Right, Left)

The Split Stance Side Stretch exercise stretches the external oblique muscles, the latissimus dorsi, and the serratus anterior muscle.

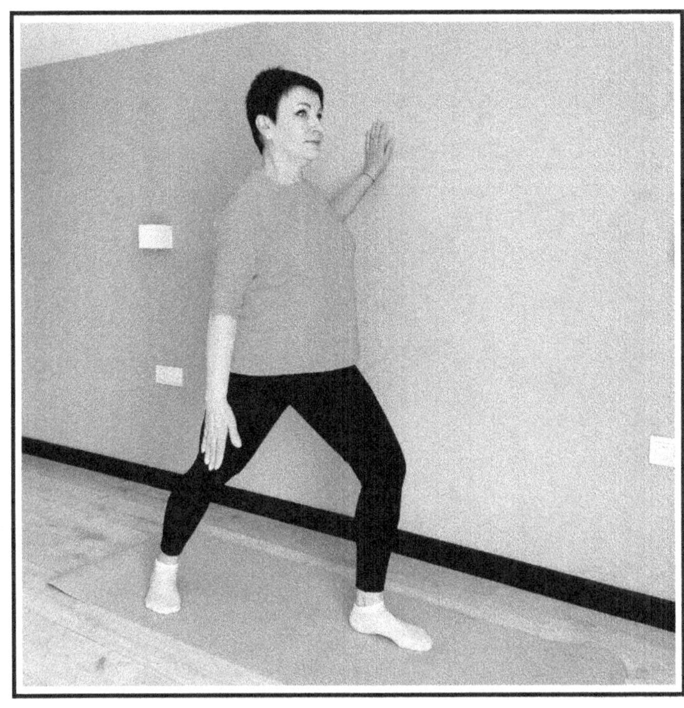

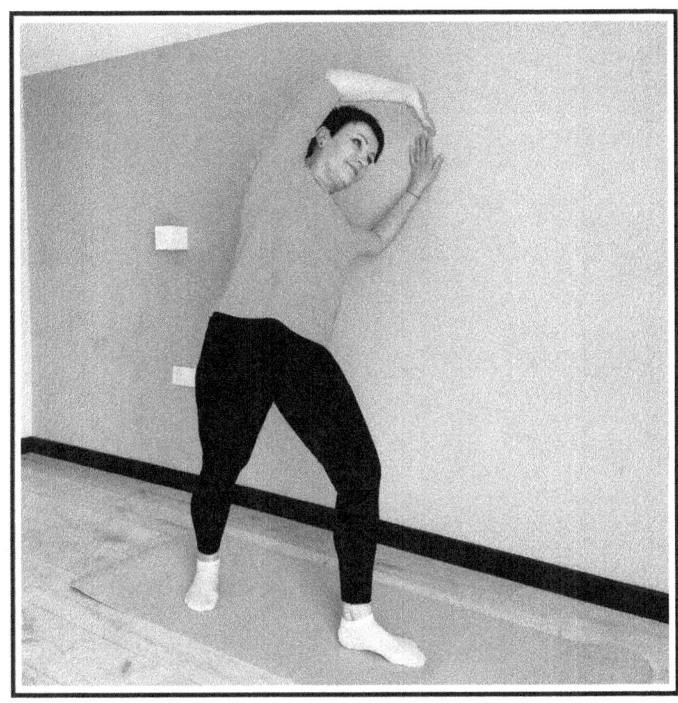

PROCEDURE:

1. Stand up tall, sideways to the wall
2. Place the left hand on the wall
3. Place the left foot forward; bring the right leg backward
4. Life the right arm upward, over the head
5. Bend gently to the left side
6. Hold the static position
7. Perform the same exercise on the opposite side

SUGGESTED TIPS:

- Try not to bend the arms
- Continue breathing throughout the exercise
- Don't move too quickly
- At the beginning of the exercise, inhale; as you lean to the side, exhale

55

Wall Back Stretch (Right, Left)

The Wall Back Stretch exercise stretches the quadratus lumborum muscle and latissimus dorsi. The exercise is highly recommended, if you have tightness in your back.

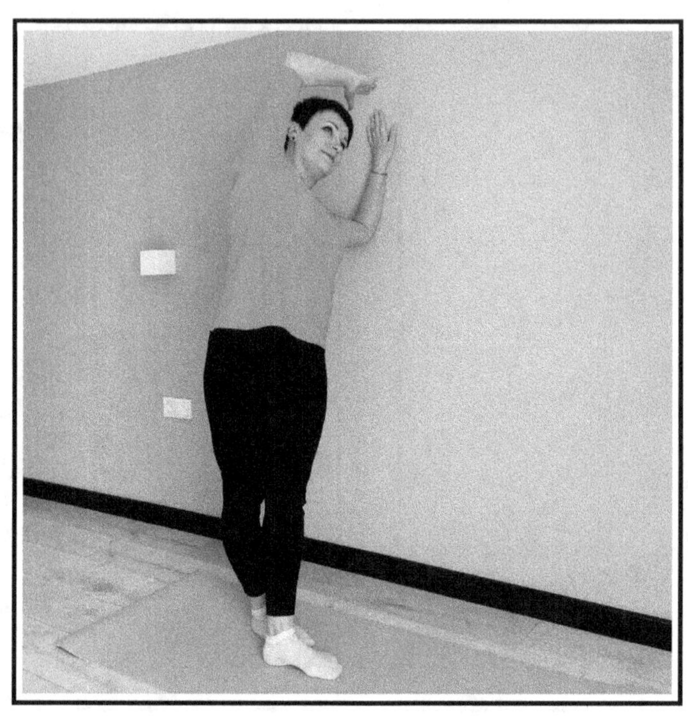

PROCEDURE:

1. Stand sideways to the wall; place the feet together
2. Place the left arm on the wall, and bend it at a 90-degree angle
3. Cross the left leg over the right leg
4. Move the right arm up and across the head
5. Hold the stretch
6. Perform the same exercise on the opposite side

SUGGESTED TIPS:

- Don't bend the knees
- Continue breathing throughout the exercise
- At the beginning of the exercise, inhale; as you continue the exercise, exhale slowly

PAGE 76

Standing Forward Bends

The Standing Forward Bends exercise is a great way to stretch the lower and upper back along with the hamstrings.

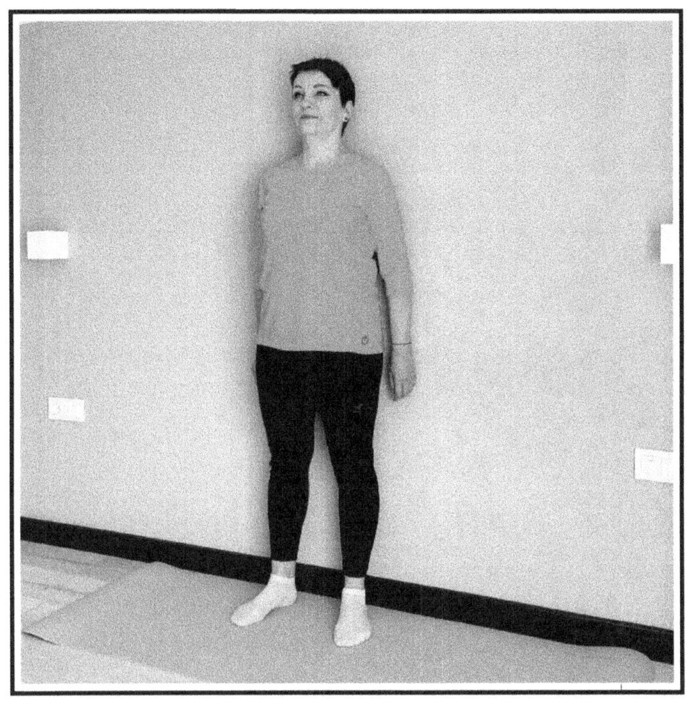 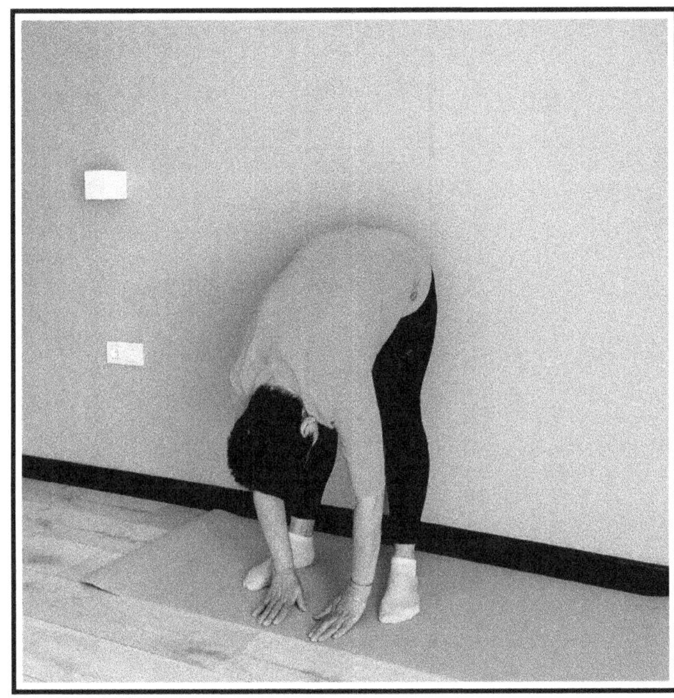

1. Stand tall hip-width apart
2. Place the glutes, upper back, and head against the wall
3. Bend the knees gently
4. Begin bending forward (round the head, upper back, and lower back)
5. Relax the arms toward the floor
6. Hold the stretch

SUGGESTED TIPS:

- Don't bend the knees too much
- Continue breathing throughout the exercise
- Keep the glutes against the wall
- At the beginning of the exercise, inhale; as you bend forward, slowly exhale

57 Seated Forward Fold

The Seated Forward Fold exercise stretches the calves and hamstring muscles and mobilizes the lower and upper back.

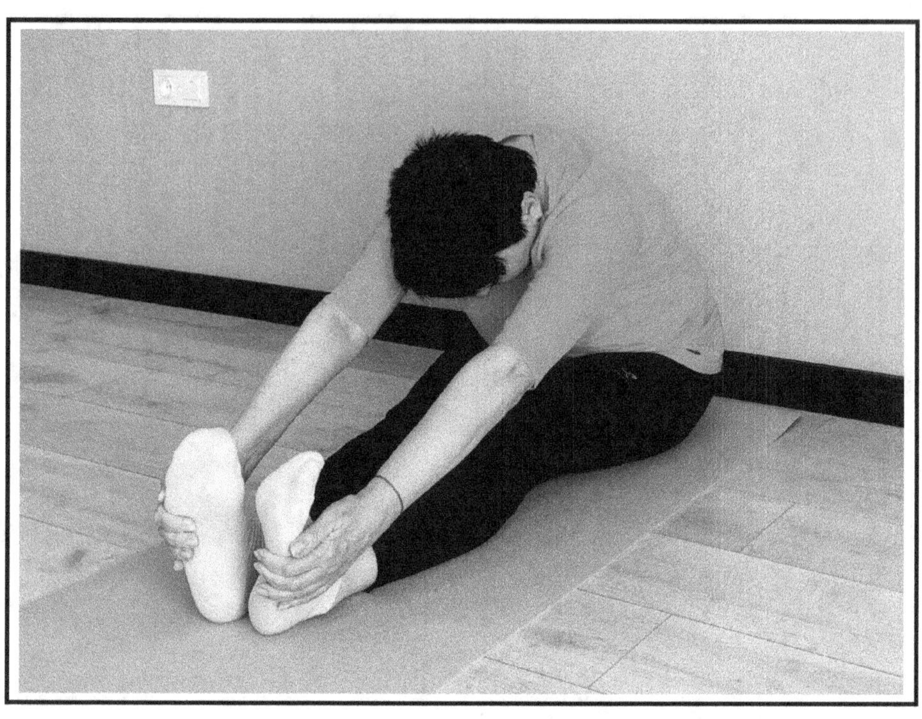

PROCEDURE:

1. Sit up tall against the wall
2. Keep the arms on the thighs
3. Keep the legs extended and bring together
4. Bend the body forward until you can touch the ankles with the fingers
5. Hold the static stretch

SUGGESTED TIPS:

- Use the full range of movement (unless you are lacking flexibility in hamstrings or lower back – then reduce the range of motion)
- Don't bend the arms or legs
- Continue breathing throughout the exercise

Child's Pose

The Child's Pose exercise can help relieve back pain and gently stretch the thighs, hips, back, and ankles.

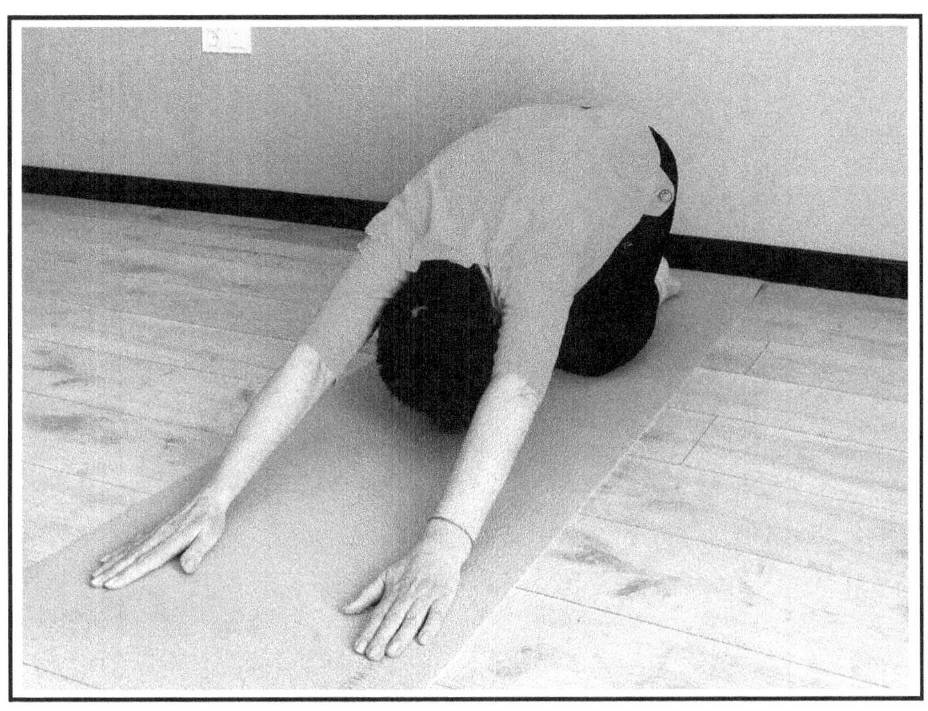

PROCEDURE:

1. Spread the knees wide, keeping the tops of your feet on the floor with the big toes touching
2. Bring the belly to rest on the floor between the forehead and thighs
3. Either stretch the arms in front of you with palms toward the floor or bring the arms back alongside your thighs with the palms facing upward
4. Remain in the position as long as you like; reconnect with the steady inhale of your breathing

SUGGESTED TIPS:

- Don't bend the neck; keep in a neutral position (use a pillow if needed)
- Avoid the exercise if you have a knee injury. Keep the arms by the side to provide support if you have a shoulder injury.

59 Wall Down Dog

The Wall Down Dog is a perfect fit to decompress the lower back and stretch the hamstrings.

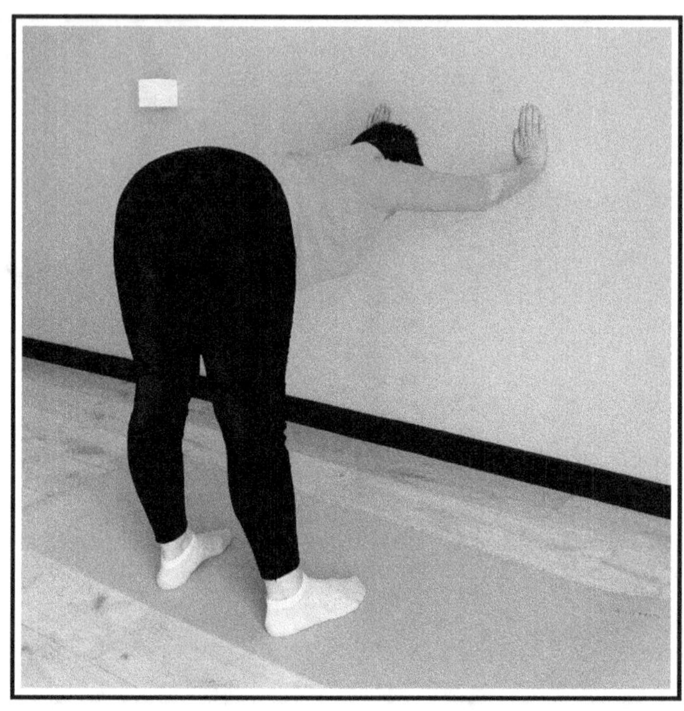

PROCEDURE:

1. Stand with the feet wider than shoulder-width apart
2. Push the hips backward and lean the hands on the wall
3. Drop the head and chest between the arms
4. Have the torso parallel to the floor
5. Hold the stretch

SUGGESTED TIPS:

- Don't bend the legs or arms
- Continue breathing throughout the exercise
- Don't arch the lower back
- At the beginning of the exercise, inhale; when you are parallel to the floor, slowly exhale

Shoulder Mobility Wall Stretch

The Shoulder Mobility Wall Stretch exercise is great for stretching the hamstrings and latissimus dorsi muscle. In addition to stretching benefits, the exercise can improve the range of shoulder motion.

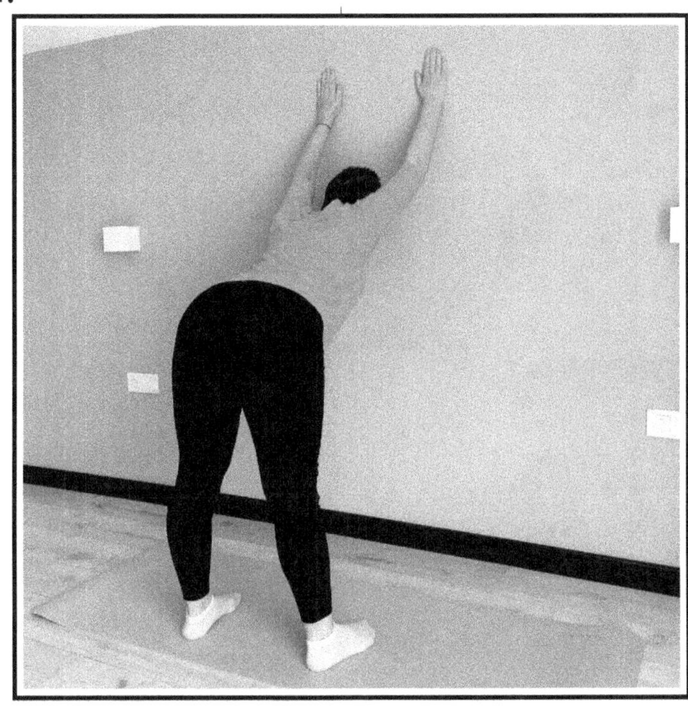

PROCEDURE:

1. Stand up tall with the feet close together
2. Place the hands on the wall (shoulder-width apart)
3. Drop the chest and push the hips backward gently
4. Hold the stretch

SUGGESTED TIPS:

- Don't bend the legs
- Don't bend the arms
- Don't arch the lower back
- Before beginning the stretch, take a deep breath; then slowly exhale through the mouth until the abdominals contract (you should feel them)

Wall Straddle Stretch

The Wall Straddle Stretch exercise stretches the adductor muscles.

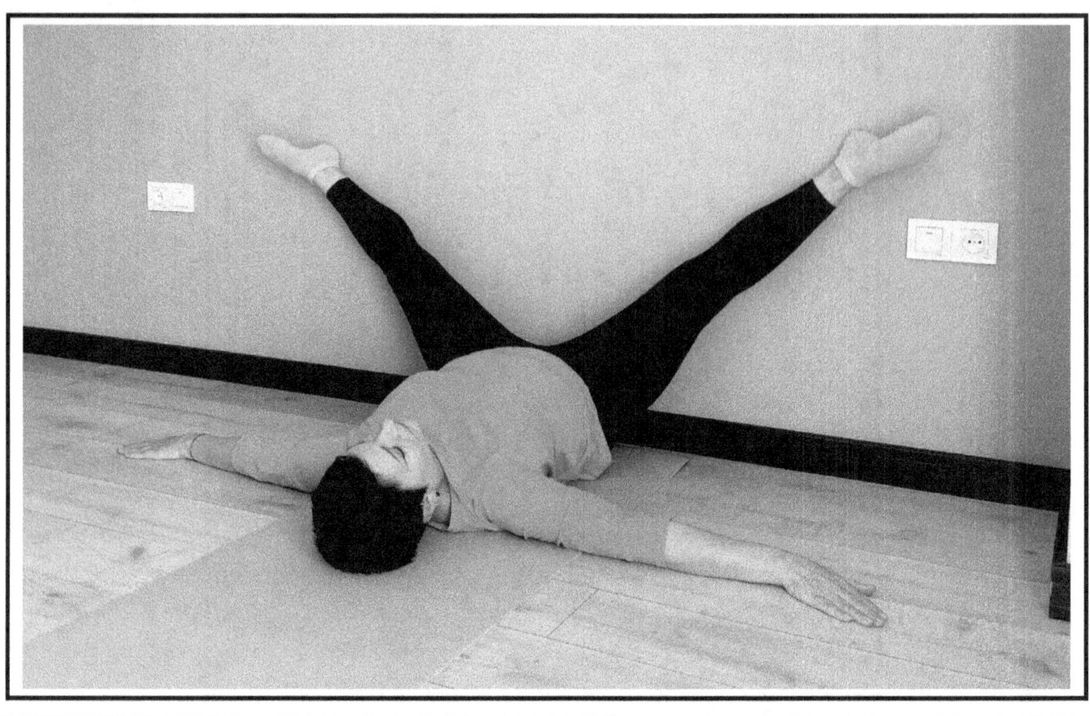

PROCEDURE:

1. Lay down flat on the back
2. Extend the legs on the wall
3. Keep the hands next to the sides
4. Straddle the legs and hold in a static position

SUGGESTED TIPS:

- Continue to breathe throughout the exercise (maintain a steady breathing pattern)
- Don't arch the lower back

Wall Frog Stretch

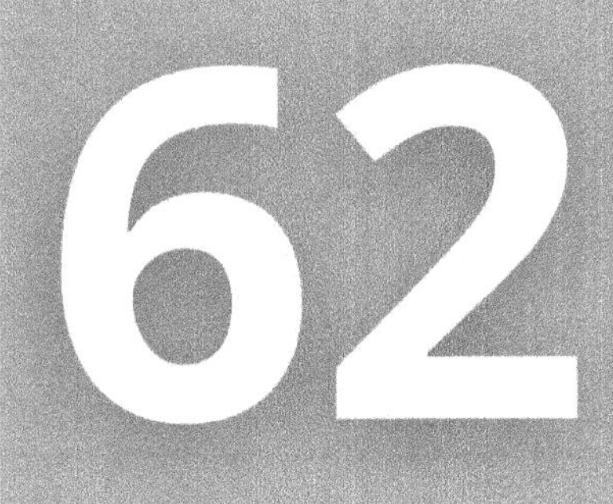

The Wall Frog Stretch works on adductor flexibility.

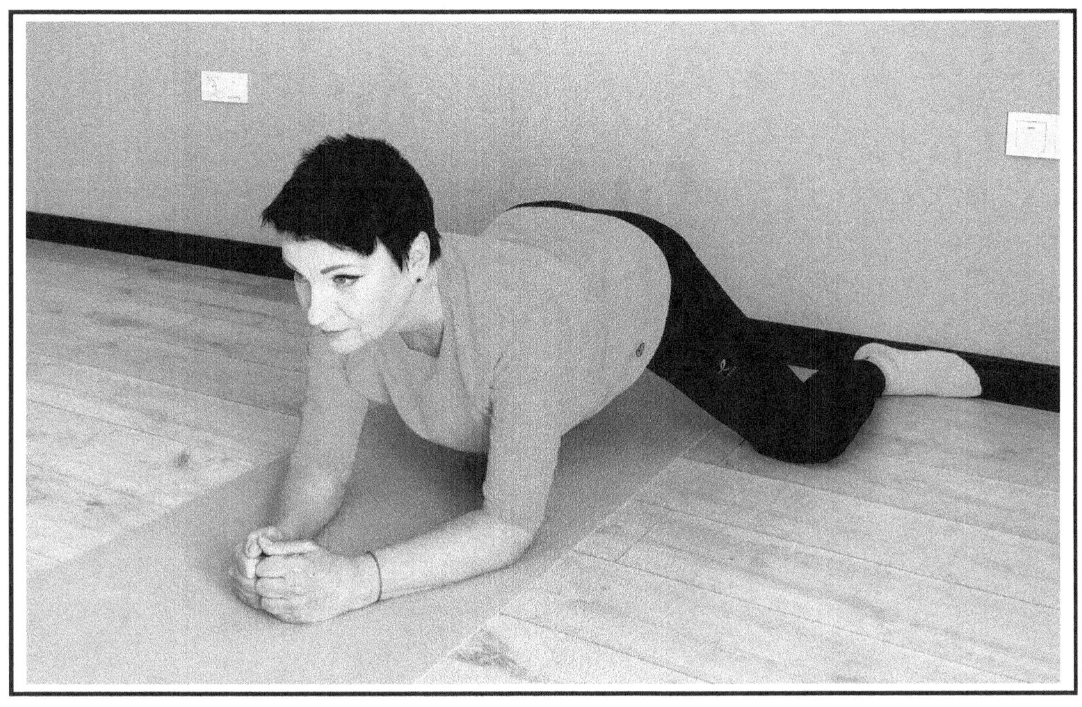

PROCEDURE:

1. Lie on your stomach
2. Rest on the elbows and knees
3. Open knees as wide as possible
4. Put the feet on the wall
5. Hold the static position

SUGGESTED TIPS:

- Don't arch the lower back
- Continue to breathe throughout the exercise (maintain a steady breathing pattern)

Butterfly Stretch

The Butterfly Stretch exercise dynamically stretches the adductor muscles.

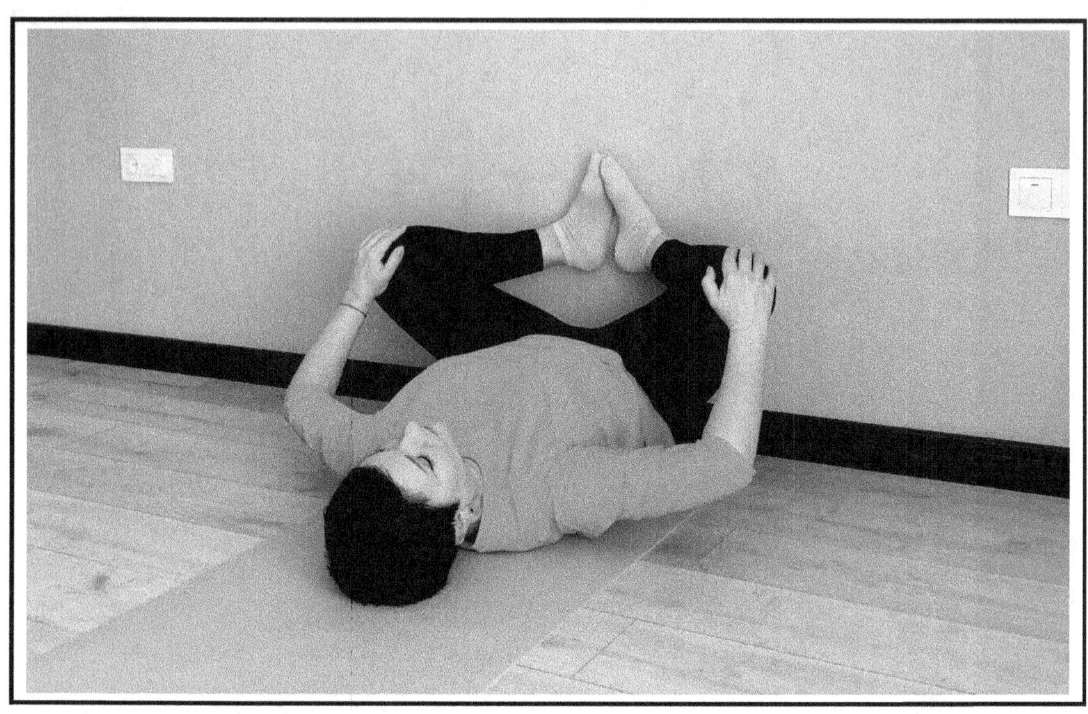

PROCEDURE:

1. Lay down flat on the back
2. Place the feet together on the wall
3. Open the hips and put your hands on them
4. Move the hands to gently press down on the knees
5. Slowly go back up
6. Repeat the exercise

SUGGESTED TIPS:

- Don't arch the lower back
- Continue to breathe throughout the exercise (maintain a steady breathing pattern)
- Don't press too hard

Reverse Frog Stretch

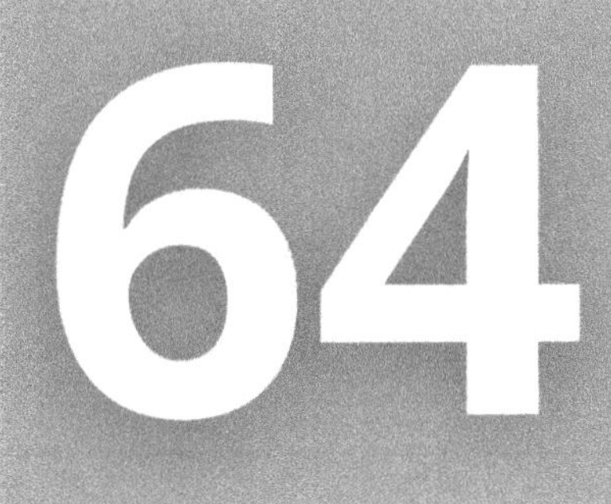

The Reverse Frog Stretch stretches the adductor muscles and is a wonderful static stretch exercise. If you feel any stiffness on the inside parts of the leg, this exercise is worth a try!

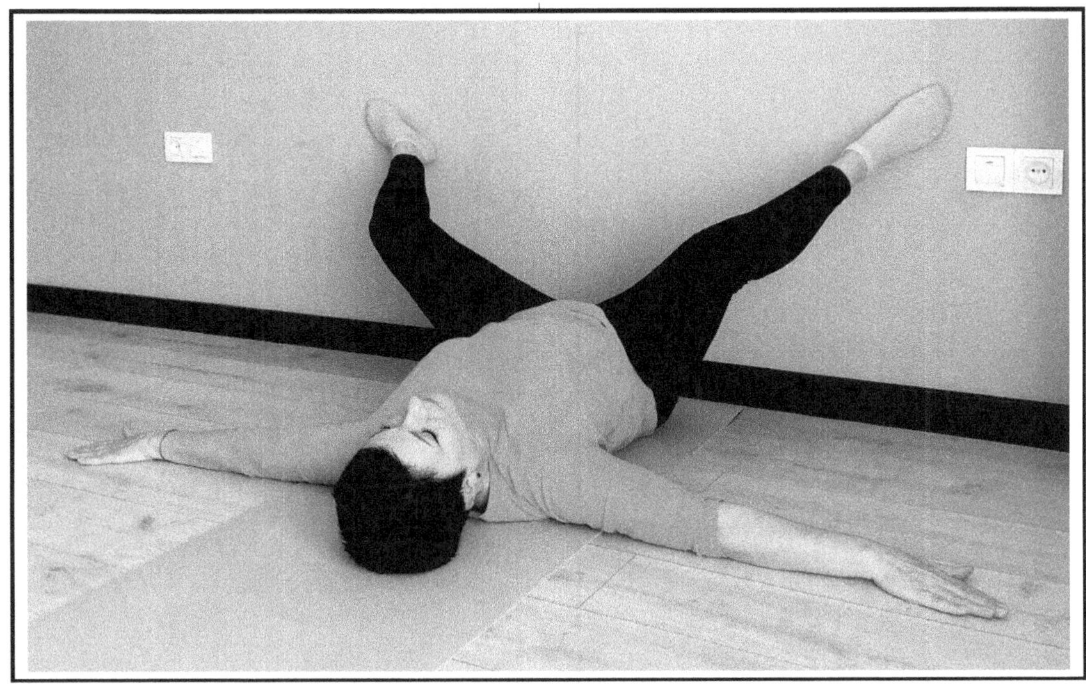

PROCEDURE:

1. Lay down flat on the back
2. Bend your knees; place the feet at a wide stance on the wall
3. Extend the arms next to the sides
4. Hold the static position

SUGGESTED TIPS:

- Don't arch the lower back
- Continue to breathe throughout the exercise (maintain a steady breathing pattern)

65 Active Frog Stretch

The Active Frog Stretch is a dynamic stretch exercise for the adductor muscles.

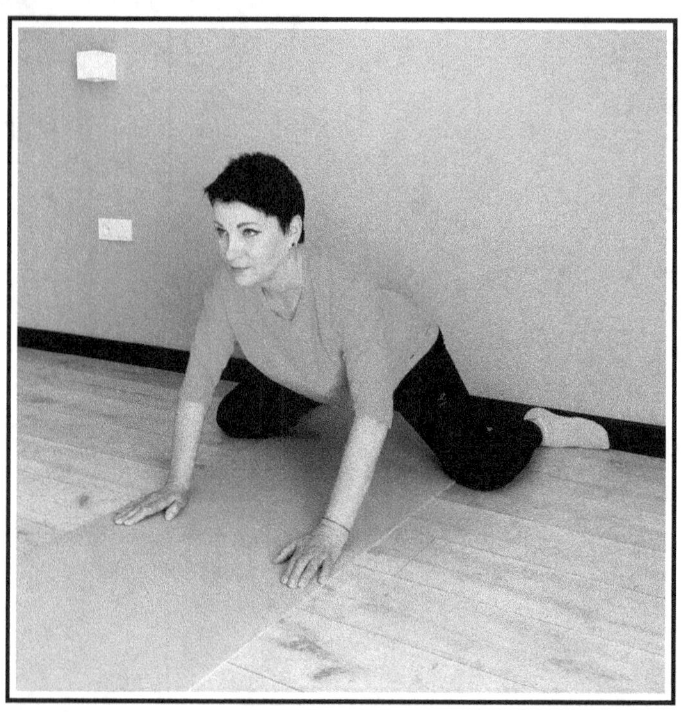 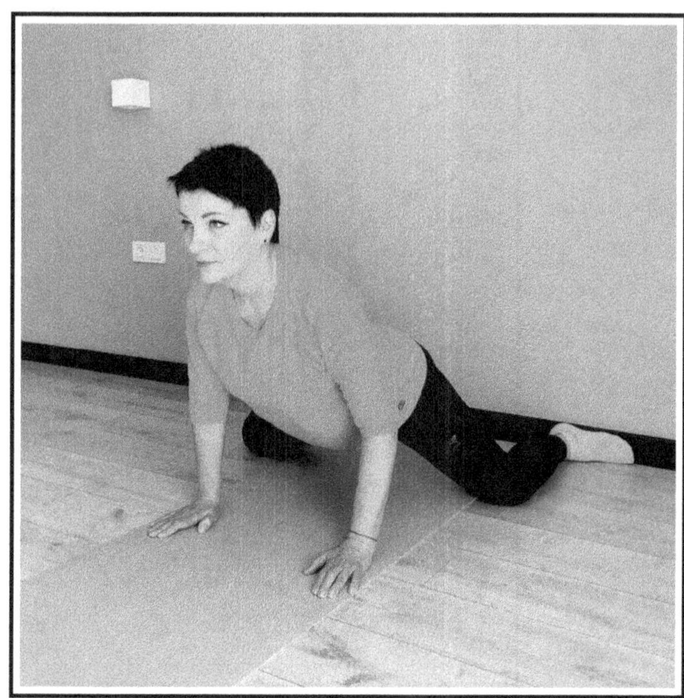

PROCEDURE:

1. Start on the floor, resting on hands
2. Open the knees as wide as possible
3. Place the feet on the wall
4. Rock the body forward and backward

SUGGESTED TIPS:

- Keep the lower back straight
- Keep the knees wide enough
- Continue to breathe throughout the exercise (maintain a steady breathing pattern)

Lying Figure 4 (Right, Left)

The Lying Figure 4 exercise works the external hip rotation. It is a wonderful exercise for hip joint health.

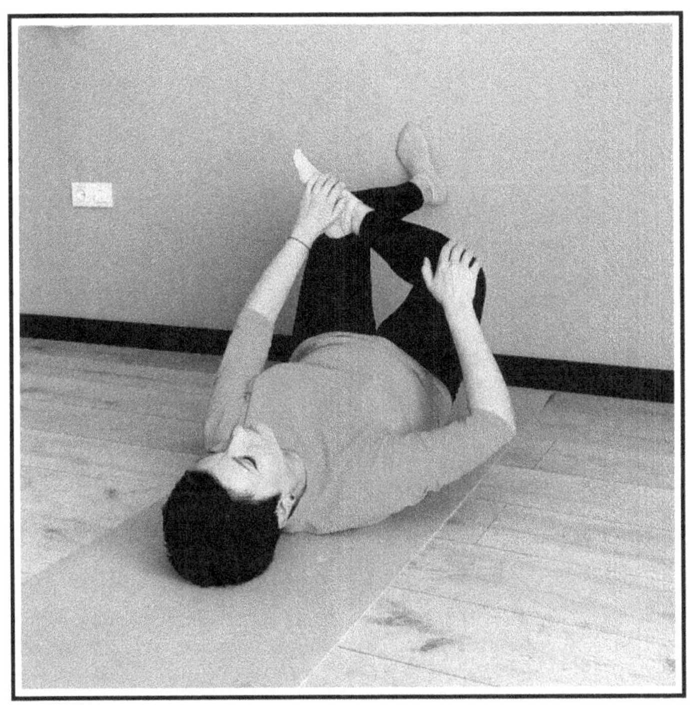
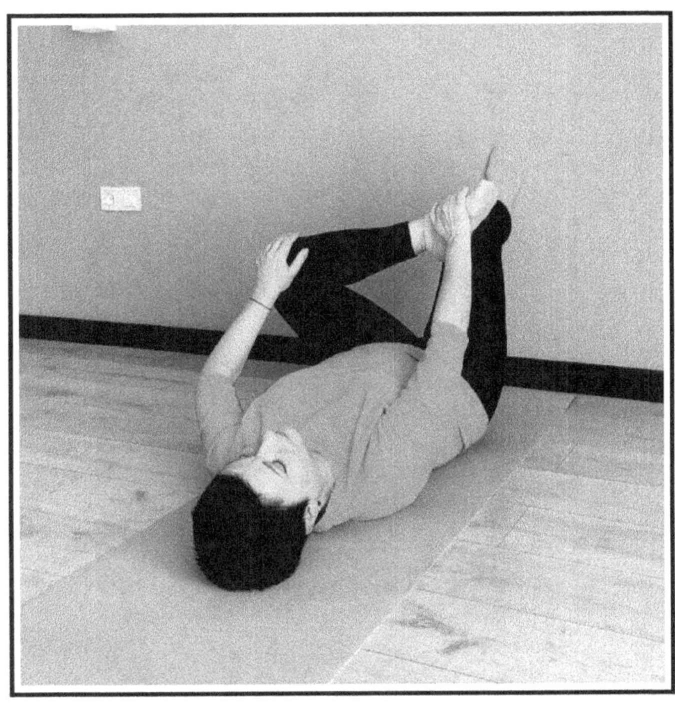

PROCEDURE:

1. Lay flat down on the back
2. Place the knees at a 90-degree angle on the wall
3. Bring the right knee to the chest
4. Grab the right ankle with the left hand
5. Rotate the right hip; place the right foot on the left knee
6. Hold the stretch; repeat with the left side

SUGGESTED TIPS:

- Let the pelvis move about
- Continue to breathe throughout the exercise (maintain a steady breathing pattern)
- Don't arch the lower back

67 Knee to Chest Stretch
(Right, Left)

The Knee to Chest Stretch exercise stretches the glute muscles and activates the hip flexor muscles.

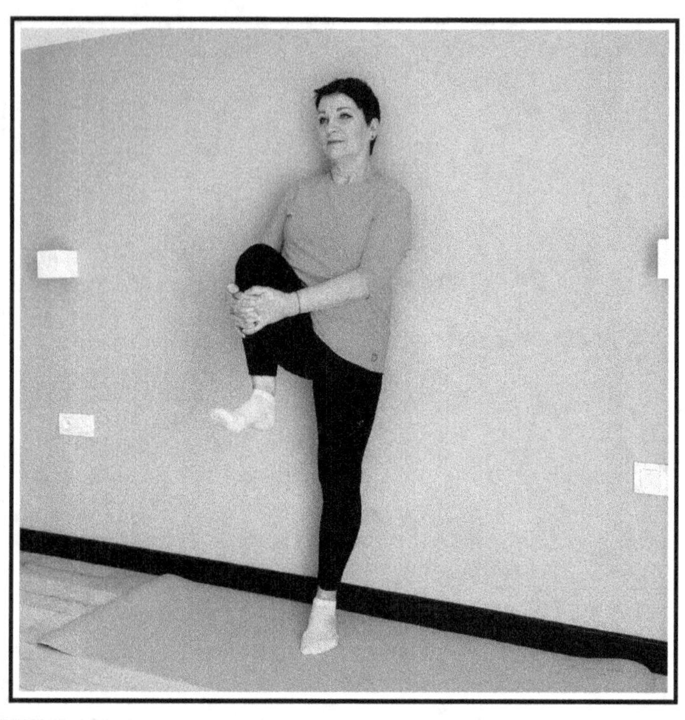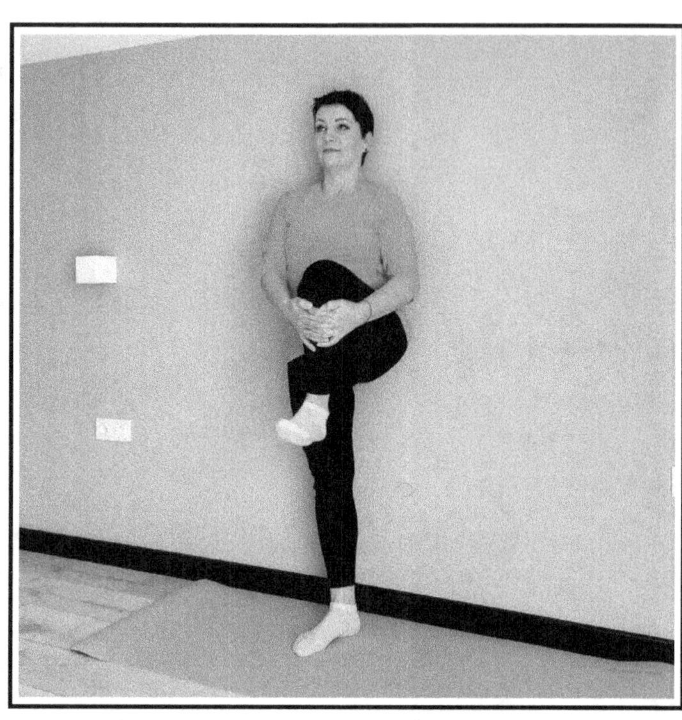

PROCEDURE:

1. Stand up tall against the wall
2. Grab the right knee; bring it toward the chest
3. Hold position; repeat with the left knee

SUGGESTED TIPS:

- Don't arch the lower back
- Don't go too fast
- Remember to hold the position
- To prevent the lower back from arching, engage the abdominal muscles prior to bringing the knees toward the chest

PAGE 88

Wall-Supported Calf Stretch (Right, Left)

The Wall-Supported Calf Stretch exercise is a great way to relax the calf muscle. No other stretch compares!

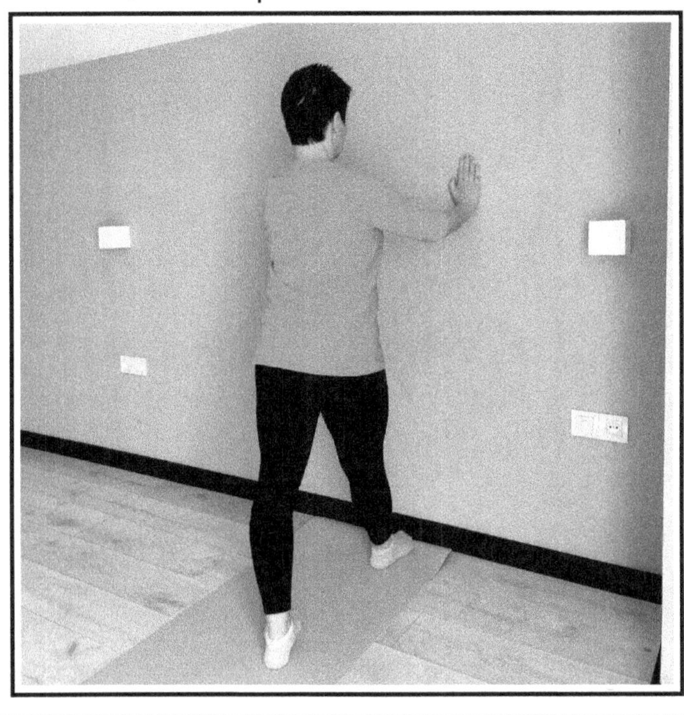
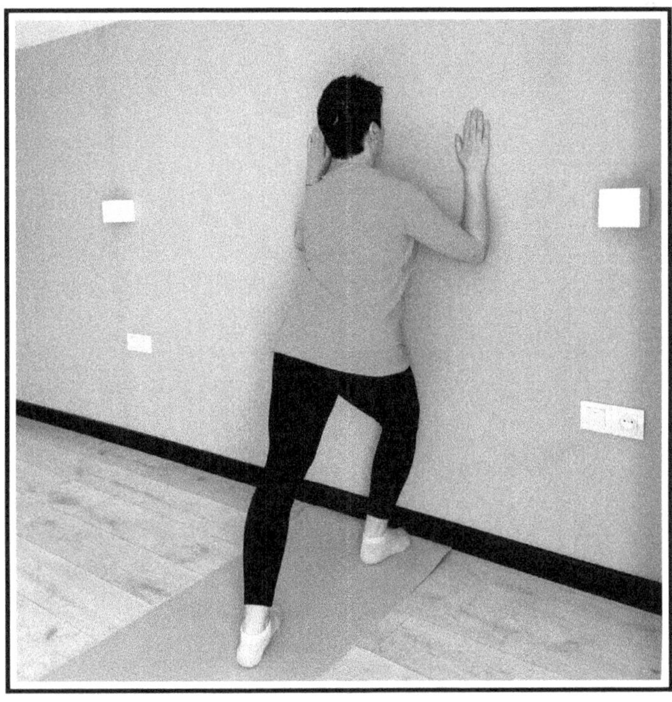

PROCEDURE:

1. Stand up tall with hands on the wall
2. Bring the right foot forward
3. Extend the left leg backward
4. Lean toward the wall by bending the right leg
5. Lean forward until you feel the stretch in the left calf muscle
6. Hold the stretch
7. Repeat with the left foot forward and right leg backward

SUGGESTED TIPS:

- Don't bend both legs
- Don't go too fast
- Bring the left foot back as far as possible to maximize the stretch

Active Calf Stretch
(Right, Left)

The Active Calf Stretch stretches the hamstrings and calves. If you are feeling some stiffness in the calves, this exercise is a must!

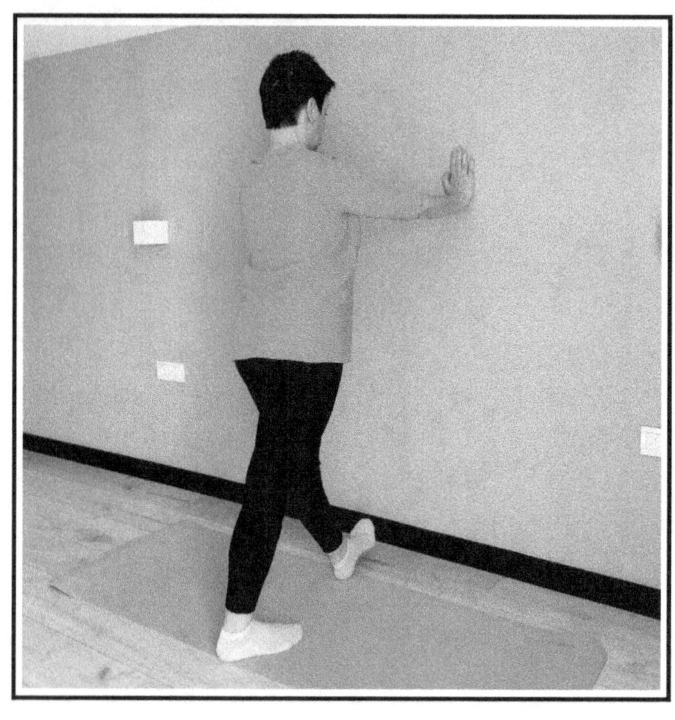 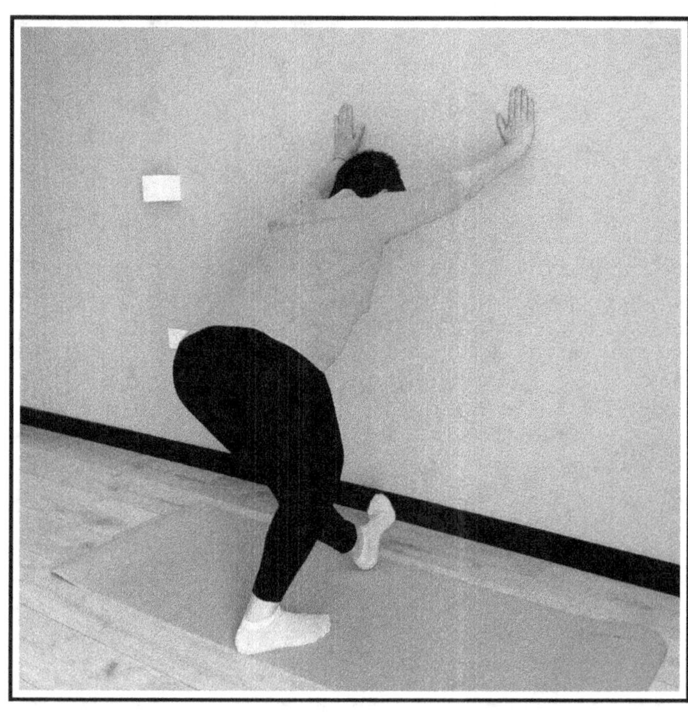

PROCEDURE:

1. Stand with the left foot in the back and the right foot forward
2. Place the hands on the wall
3. Bend the left knee; bring the right toes up
4. Extend back to the previous position; repeat the movement
5. Perform the same exercise with the opposite foot and knee

SUGGESTED TIPS:

- Don't hold your breath
- Don't rush through the exercise
- Don't bend both legs in every step of the exercise
- To increase the stretch, hold the static contraction longer

Spinal Twist
(Right, Left)

The Spinal Twist exercise is a great one to use for stretching the lower back perfectly.

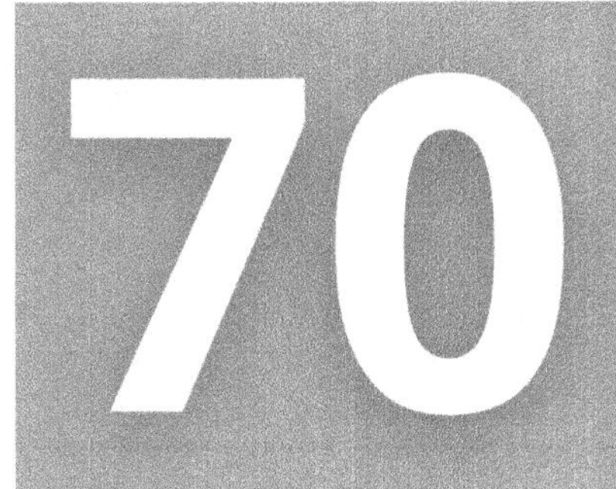

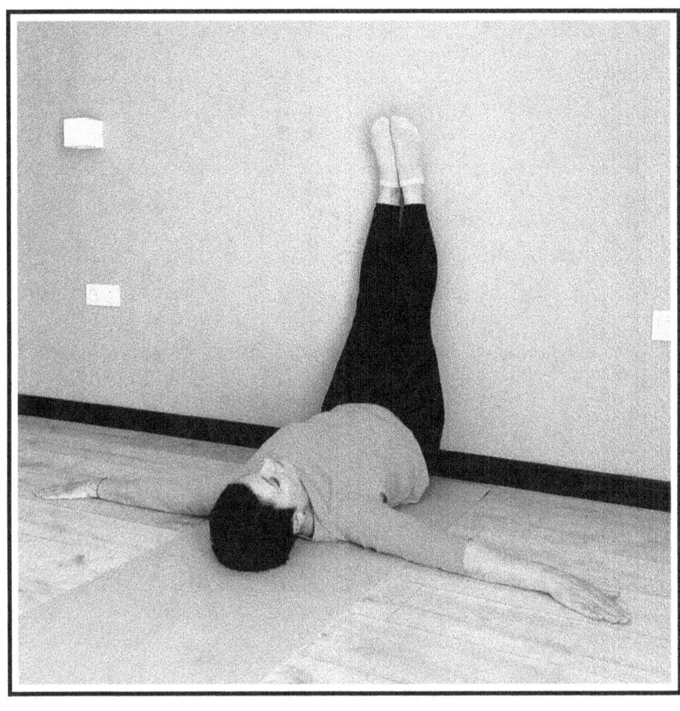

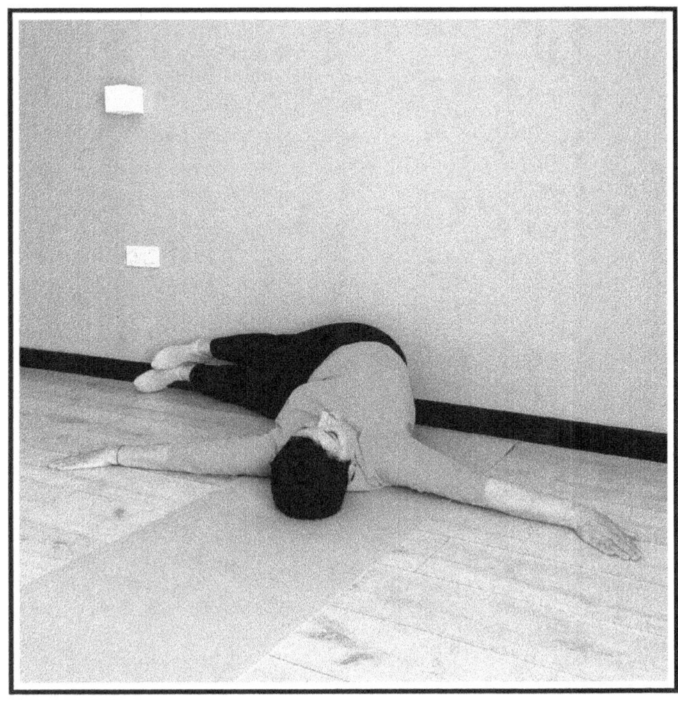

1. Lay down flat on the back
2. Extend the legs on the wall
3. Keep the hands next to the sides
4. Bring the legs down (slowly and with control) to the right side
5. Hold position
6. Repeat to the left side

- Don't bend the knees
- Keep breathing throughout the exercise
- To increase stretch effectiveness, breathe through the stomach area

28-Day Workout Challenge

DAY 1
Full Body

WARM-UP
6 - 30/30 sec
2 - 30 sec
10 - 30 sec

MAIN WORKOUT
12 - 40 sec
26 - 40 sec
43 - 40 sec
29 - 40 sec
35 - 40 sec

STRETCHING
68 - 30/30 sec
65 - 30 sec
54 - 30/30 sec

DAY 2
Arms, Chest, Back

WARM-UP
8 - 30 sec
4 - 30 sec
6 - 30/30 sec

MAIN WORKOUT
22 - 40 sec
35 - 40 sec
38 - 40 sec
40 - 40 sec
39 - 40 sec

STRETCHING
50 - 30 sec
51 - 30 sec
54 - 30/30 sec

DAY 3
Full Body

WARM-UP
3 - 30/30 sec
11 - 30 sec
7 - 30/30 sec

MAIN WORKOUT
13 - 40 sec
44 - 40 sec
48 - 40/40 sec
30 - 40 sec
37 - 40 sec

STRETCHING
69 - 30/30 sec
63 - 30 sec
50 - 30 sec

DAY 4
Legs, Glutes

WARM-UP
9 - 30 sec
1 - 30/30 sec
5 - 30 sec

MAIN WORKOUT
18 - 40 sec
27 - 40/40 sec
13 - 40 sec
15 - 40 sec
22 - 40 sec

STRETCHING
61 - 30 sec
66 - 30/30 sec
68 - 30 sec

DAY 5
Full Body

WARM-UP
6 - 30/30 sec
2 - 30 sec
10 - 30 sec

MAIN WORKOUT
14 - 40/40 sec
45 - 40 sec
20 - 40 sec
31 - 40 sec
38 - 40 sec

STRETCHING
67 - 30/30 sec
62 - 30 sec
55 - 30/30 sec

DAY 6
Belly

WARM-UP
8 - 30 sec
4 - 30 sec
6 - 30/30 sec

MAIN WORKOUT
23 - 40/40 sec
29 - 40 sec
31 - 40 sec
32 - 40 sec
24 - 40/40 sec

STRETCHING
60 - 30 sec
70 - 30/30 sec
57 - 30 sec

Take a 15-30 second break between exercises, depending on how you feel, to allow your body to recover and maintain optimal performance

DAY 7
DAY OFF

DAY 8
Full Body

WARM-UP
3 - 30/30 sec
11 - 30 sec
7 - 30/30 sec

MAIN WORKOUT
15 - 40 sec
24 - 40/40 sec
47 - 40/40 sec
34 - 40 sec
39 - 40 sec

STRETCHING
56 - 30 sec
49 - 30/30 sec
63 - 30 sec

DAY 9
Arms, Chest, Back

WARM-UP
9 - 30 sec
1 - 30/30 sec
5 - 30 sec

MAIN WORKOUT
21 - 40 sec
36 - 40 sec
37 - 40 sec
41 - 40 sec
42 - 40 sec

STRETCHING
52 - 30 sec
53 - 30 sec
58 - 30 sec

DAY 10
Full Body

WARM-UP
6 - 30/30 sec
2 - 30 sec
10 - 30 sec

MAIN WORKOUT
16 - 40 sec
25 - 40 sec
17 - 40 sec
18 - 40 sec
32 - 40 sec

STRETCHING
68 - 30/30 sec
65 - 30 sec
54 - 30/30 sec

DAY 11
Legs, Glutes

WARM-UP
8 - 30 sec
4 - 30 sec
6 - 30/30 sec

MAIN WORKOUT
19 - 40 sec
28 - 40 sec
12 - 40 sec
16 - 40 sec
21 - 40 sec

STRETCHING
64 - 30 sec
67 - 30/30 sec
69 - 30/30 sec

DAY 12
Full Body

WARM-UP
3 - 30/30 sec
11 - 30 sec
7 - 30/30 sec

MAIN WORKOUT
17 - 40 sec
46 - 40 sec
19 - 40 sec
23 - 40/40 sec
33 - 40 sec

STRETCHING
69 - 30/30 sec
63 - 30 sec
50 - 30 sec

DAY 13
Belly

WARM-UP
9 - 30 sec
1 - 30/30 sec
5 - 30 sec

MAIN WORKOUT
20 - 40 sec
30 - 40 sec
34 - 40 sec
33 - 40 sec
14 - 40/40 sec

STRETCHING
55 - 30/30 sec
59 - 30 sec
70 - 30/30 sec

Take a 15-30 second break between exercises, depending on how you feel, to allow your body to recover and maintain optimal performance

DAY 7
DAY OFF

DAY 15
Full Body

WARM-UP
6 - 30/30 sec
2 - 30 sec
10 - 30 sec

MAIN WORKOUT
12 - 50 sec
26 - 50 sec
43 - 50 sec
29 - 50 sec
35 - 50 sec

STRETCHING
68 - 30/30 sec
65 - 30 sec
54 - 30/30 sec

DAY 16
Arms, Chest, Back

WARM-UP
8 - 30 sec
4 - 30 sec
6 - 30/30 sec

MAIN WORKOUT
22 - 50 sec
35 - 50 sec
38 - 50 sec
40 - 50 sec
39 - 50 sec

STRETCHING
50 - 30 sec
51 - 30 sec
54 - 30/30 sec

DAY 17
Full Body

WARM-UP
3 - 30/30 sec
11 - 30 sec
7 - 30/30 sec

MAIN WORKOUT
13 - 50 sec
44 - 50 sec
48 - 50/50 sec
30 - 50 sec
37 - 50 sec

STRETCHING
69 - 30/30 sec
63 - 30 sec
50 - 30 sec

DAY 18
Legs, Glutes

WARM-UP
9 - 30 sec
1 - 30/30 sec
5 - 30 sec

MAIN WORKOUT
18 - 50 sec
27 - 50/50 sec
13 - 50 sec
15 - 50 sec
22 - 50 sec

STRETCHING
61 - 30 sec
66 - 30/30 sec
68 - 30 sec

DAY 19
Full Body

WARM-UP
6 - 30/30 sec
2 - 30 sec
10 - 30 sec

MAIN WORKOUT
14 - 50/50 sec
45 - 50 sec
20 - 50 sec
31 - 50 sec
38 - 50 sec

STRETCHING
67 - 30/30 sec
62 - 30 sec
55 - 30/30 sec

DAY 20
Belly

WARM-UP
8 - 30 sec
4 - 30 sec
6 - 30/30 sec

MAIN WORKOUT
23 - 50/50 sec
29 - 50 sec
31 - 50 sec
32 - 50 sec
24 - 50/50 sec

STRETCHING
60 - 30 sec
70 - 30/30 sec
57 - 30 sec

Take a 15-30 second break between exercises, depending on how you feel, to allow your body to recover and maintain optimal performance

DAY 7
DAY OFF

DAY 22
Full Body

WARM-UP
3 - 30/30 sec
11 - 30 sec
7 - 30/30 sec

MAIN WORKOUT
15 - 50 sec
24 - 50/50 sec
47 - 50/50 sec
34 - 50 sec
39 - 50 sec
#48 - 50 sec

STRETCHING
56 - 30 sec
49 - 30/30 sec
63 - 30 sec

DAY 23
Arms, Chest, Back

WARM-UP
9 - 30 sec
1 - 30/30 sec
5 - 30 sec

MAIN WORKOUT
21 - 50 sec
36 - 50 sec
37 - 50 sec
41 - 50 sec
42 - 50 sec
28 - 50 sec

STRETCHING
52 - 30 sec
53 - 30 sec
58 - 30 sec

DAY 24
Full Body

WARM-UP
6 - 30/30 sec
2 - 30 sec
10 - 30 sec

MAIN WORKOUT
16 - 50 sec
25 - 50 sec
17 - 50 sec
18 - 50 sec
32 - 50 sec
44 - 50 sec

STRETCHING
68 - 30/30 sec
65 - 30 sec
54 - 30/30 sec

DAY 25
Legs, Glutes

WARM-UP
8 - 30 sec
4 - 30 sec
6 - 30/30 sec

MAIN WORKOUT
19 - 50 sec
28 - 50 sec
12 - 50 sec
16 - 50 sec
21 - 50 sec
25 - 50 sec

STRETCHING
64 - 30 sec
67 - 30/30 sec
69 - 30/30 sec

DAY 26
Full Body

WARM-UP
3 - 30/30 sec
11 - 30 sec
7 - 30/30 sec

MAIN WORKOUT
17 - 50 sec
46 - 50 sec
19 - 50 sec
23 - 50/50 sec
33 - 50 sec
26 - 50 sec

STRETCHING
69 - 30/30 sec
63 - 30 sec
50 - 30 sec

DAY 27
Belly

WARM-UP
9 - 30 sec
1 - 30/30 sec
5 - 30 sec

MAIN WORKOUT
20 - 50 sec
30 - 50 sec
34 - 50 sec
33 - 50 sec
14 - 50/50 sec
27 - 50 sec

STRETCHING
55 - 30/30 sec
59 - 30 sec
70 - 30/30 sec

Take a 15-30 second break between exercises, depending on how you feel, to allow your body to recover and maintain optimal performance

DAY 7
DAY OFF

Conclusion

Wall Pilates for Seniors by FitLife Solutions has given you a comprehensive path to reaching your fitness goals. Throughout this journey, you have learned many valuable insights, effective workout techniques, and practical tips that will help you lead a happier, healthier life.

With the tools and knowledge gained, you can succeed! Just apply what you have learned to your daily life, one step at a time. No matter if you are striving for weight loss, balance, strength, or overall wellness, you have the power to create a positive change in your life.

We want to thank you for coming along with us on this transformative journey. We wish you a future filled with vitality, health, and limitless energy. Keep progressing and, remember, fitness success begins with you!

References

- Ackler, M. (2023, July 28). What is Wall Pilates? Pilates Anytime. https://www.pilatesanytime.com/blog/equipment/what-is-wall-pilates

- Better Me Pilates: Pilates at Home. (n.d.). Better Me. https://betterme.world

- Geoghegan, C. (2023, Sept. 4). A Beginner Guide to Wall Pilates: Everything You Need to Know as a Runner. Run with Caroline. https://www.runwithcaroline.com/wall-pilates/

- Hardy, L. (2023, July 14). Wall Pilates Exercises for Seniors. Wall Pilates. https://wallpilates.com/wall-pilates-exercises-for-seniors/

- Learn How to Get a Healthier Life with Pilates and Chiropractic Care. (2023, June 15). Prestige Health and Wellness. https://www.prestigehealthwellness.com/unlocking-the-power-of-pilates-a-path-to-a-healthier-lifestyle-for-chiropractic-care-enthusiasts/

- The Evolution of Pilates Equipment: Past, Present, and Future Trends. (2023, Dec. 25). Pilates Reformers Plus. https://pilatesreformersplus.com/blogs/news/the-evolution-of-pilates-equipment-past-present-and-future-trends

- What Is Diaphragmatic Breathing? (2023, May 19). Healthline. https://www.healthline.com/health/diaphragmatic-breathing